Video Casebook: Medicine

Video Casebook: Medicine

The toy boy and the burgundy car

Andrew Levy PhD FRCP

University of Bristol, Department of Medicine Laboratories,
Bristol Royal Infirmary, Lower Maudlin Street,
Bristol BS2 8HW, UK

Blackwell
Science

Editorial Offices:
Osney Mead, Oxford OX2 0EL
25 John Street, London WC1N 2BL
23 Ainslie Place, Edinburgh EH3 6AJ
350 Main Street, Malden
MA 02148-5018, USA
54 University Street, Carlton
Victoria 3053, Australia
10, rue Casimir Delavigne
75006 Paris, France

Other Editorial Offices:
Blackwell Wissenschafts-Verlag GmbH
Kurfürstendamm 57
10707 Berlin, Germany

Blackwell Science KK
MG Kodenmacho Building
7–10 Kodenmacho Nihombashi
Chuo-ku, Tokyo 104, Japan

First published 1999

Set by Excel Typesetters Co., Hong Kong
Printed and bound in Great Britain at the Alden Press Ltd, Oxford and Northampton

DISTRIBUTORS

Marston Book Services Ltd
PO Box 269
Abingdon, Oxon OX14 4YN
(*Orders*: Tel: 01235 465500
Fax: 01235 465555)

USA
Blackwell Science, Inc.
Commerce Place
350 Main Street
Malden, MA 02148-5018
(*Orders*: Tel: 800 759 6102
781 388 8250
Fax: 781 388 8255)

Canada
Login Brothers Book Company
324 Saulteaux Crescent
Winnipeg, Manitoba R3J 3T2
(*Orders*: Tel: 204 837-2987)

Australia
Blackwell Science Pty Ltd
54 University Street
Carlton, Victoria 3053
(*Orders*: Tel: 3 9347 0300
Fax: 3 9347 5001)

A catalogue record for this title is available from the British Library

ISBN 0-632-05122-1

Library of Congress
Cataloging-in-publication Data

Levy, Andrew, Dr.
The toy boy and the burgundy car / Andrew Levy.
p. cm.—(Video casebook: medicine)
ISBN 0-632-05122-1
1. Internal medicine Case studies. I. Title.
II. Series.
[DNLM: 1. Diagnostic Techniques and Procedures Case Report.
2. Diagnostic Techniques and Procedures Problems and Exercises. WB 18.2 L668t 1999]
RC66.L39—1999
616.07′5—dc21
DNLM/DLC
for Library of Congress 99-21518
CIP

For further information on Blackwell Science, visit our website:
www.blackwell-science.com

Contents

Case Studies

Preface

The ability to unravel the nature of diseases merely by listening to patients describing their symptoms is one of the most fundamental and satisfying skills in medicine. As meeting a patient face to face is more memorable than reading about a condition in isolation, this collection of 50 case histories is accompanied by the next best thing—a unique compilation of interviews and video footage of the patients on CD-ROM.

Impromptu interviews were conducted on a one-to-one basis during out-patient consultations or after ward rounds. In each case the handheld video footage of unrehearsed interviews conveys the real clinical situation and the patients' genuine interpretation of events leading up to their presentation.

The CD does not merely duplicate the material in the accompanying text. The video and sound files are complementary and unique additions.

AL

Acknowledgements

The author would like to thank his colleagues, particularly Dr Paul Taylor at Hanham Surgery, Dr Ken Heaton, Dr Ralph Barry, Dr Graham Standon and Dr Julian Kabala all at The Bristol Royal Infirmary and Dr Charlie Tomson at Southmead Hospital for access to their patients and their bemused hospitality.

The original camcorder and video editing platform were provided by Madeleine Curtis of Bayer PLC and Sandoz PLC. Dr Mike Stein from Blackwell Science had the insight to replace the camcorder after its untimely theft.

Dedication

To the 50 magnificent patients whose spontaneous goodwill and humour made this presentation possible; to my family, Ainslie, Rebecca, Hannah and Daniel, who put up with me, and to the staff of Blackwell Science who without exception were a pleasure to work with.

Technical note

The video and sound footage, still images and text were recorded, edited, compiled and produced in a book and CD-ROM format by the author. Video material was recorded using a Sony CCD-TR750 and subsequently a Sony CCD-TR810E Hi8 camera. Hi8 sound was recorded through a Sony ECM-55 microphone. Images were digitized using a Macintosh PowerPC 8100/100 equipped with a Radius VideoVision Studio™ board, JPEG compressed in real time and written onto a 4 Gb FWB Sledgehammer™ hard disc array. Adobe Premiere 4.01™ was used for non-linear video and sound editing. Digital images were edited in Adobe Premiere and exported pict files edited with Adobe Photoshop 3.0™. Illustrations were generated using Adobe Photoshop 3.0™, Adobe Illustrator 6.0™ and MacDrawPro™ and then professionally redrawn for Blackwell Science Ltd. The CD-ROM presentation authoring programme was Macromedia Director 5.0™ on the Mac platform.

Case Studies

Case 1
The toy boy and the burgundy car

History

A 56-year-old secondary school teacher was admitted to hospital with a 3-day history of a cough productive of green sputum and increasing shortness of breath. She had previously been entirely well and, according to her relatives, had no significant past medical history. The most prominent feature of her admission was that the history had to be taken from the patient's spouse as the patient herself was completely disorientated in time, place and person. She showed marked restlessness and agitation, was unable to answer questions or cooperate in any way and was clearly having vivid and unpleasant visual hallucinations.

The findings on examination were consistent with a chest infection which responded well to treatment with antibiotics. Although her recovery from the chest infection itself was rapid and uncomplicated, her mental state remained highly unsettled with aggressive outbursts and flight of ideas that necessitated transfer to the local psychiatric hospital. After several days, what had been assumed to be an acute confusional state induced by infection was reassessed.

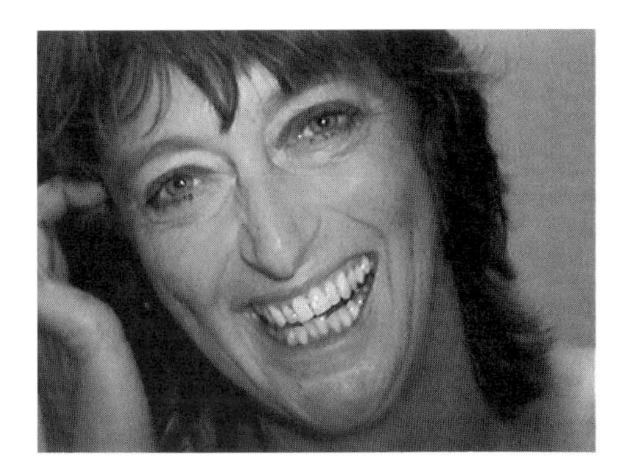

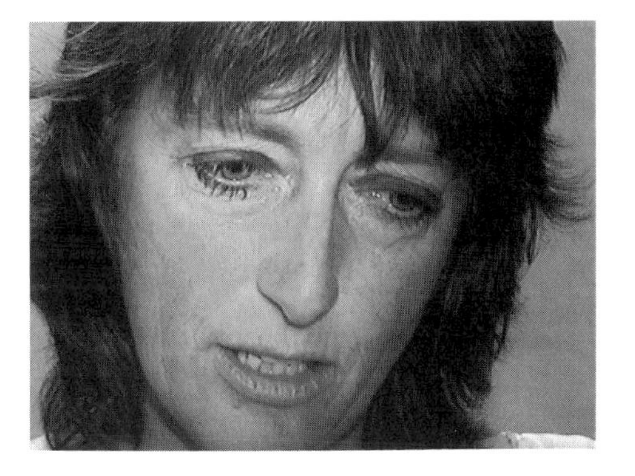

Notes

The patient had developed manic depressive psychosis.

Symptoms of depression include tearful or depressed appearance and mood, lack of changes in mood in response to environmental events, social withdrawal, markedly diminished pleasure or interest in most activities, recurrent thoughts of death or suicide and feelings of worthlessness, guilt and self-pity or pessimism. In contrast, fatigue, weight loss, symptoms of anxiety and symptoms related to the genitals are generally not associated with major depressive illness.

Depressive psychosis and bipolar illness are relatively common psychiatric syndromes. Bipolar illness, in which hypomania and depression both occur, has a mean age of onset in youth (24–32 years) and affects almost 1.5% of the population. First episodes are manic in 60% of cases, and many of these patients have conditions that remain predominantly manic in character, while 30% manifest primarily depressive disease. The rate of cycling from one to the other tends to increase with time. Concordance with monozygotic twins averages 65% and is 15% with dizygotic twins, yet attempts to identify any linkage with a variety of candidate genes have so far proven unsuccessful. The hereditary nature of the condition is reaffirmed by the **patient's story** of her friend and her friend's mother (met at group therapy), both of whom have manic depressive psychosis.

The organic nature of the condition is further demonstrated by the observation that up to 50% of depressed patients have no dexamethasone-induced suppression of adrenal cortisol production (i.e. the biochemical picture of Cushing's syndrome). Furthermore, in 35–50% of patients, the thyrotrophin response to thyrotrophin-releasing hormone is blunted.

Lithium is a classical treatment, but its efficacy may be little better than carbamazepine or sodium valproate.

Basic science

Linkage studies and seasonality

Many genes, including the γ-aminobutyric acid(A) (GABA(A)), 5-hydroxytryptamine and dopamine receptors and 5-hydroxytryptamine and dopamine transporters, have been excluded by linkage studies. Regions of chromosomes 18 and 21 have been implicated, and there has repeatedly been shown to be a 5–8% winter–spring excess of births for mania and bipolar disorder. This unexplained seasonal birth excess, which extends from December to March, is also found in schizophrenia and schizoaffective disorder. The risks of schizophrenia are not related to gender, social class, race, birth complications or the use of various diagnostic central nervous system imaging technologies. Unfortunately, at the time of writing, virtually no correlation studies have been carried out for bipolar disorder.

In relation to **other medical conditions** and circumstances, the most frequent precipitants of mania are corticosteroids and temporolimbic epilepsy, and of depression, stroke and Parkinson's disease. Human immunodeficiency virus infection has been found to be closely associated with both mania and depression.

Diseases causing depression

Hypothyroidism and hyperthyroidism
Cushing's syndrome
Systemic lupus erythematosus
Congestive cardiac failure and myocardial infarction
Multiple sclerosis (euphoria can also occur)
Hepatitis
Malignancies
Metabolic disorders, such as porphyria
Vitamin deficiencies (thiamine, nicotinic acid—pellagra)

Drugs causing depression

Corticosteroids
Reserpine

MCQs

1 Bipolar depression (depression with episodes of mania) is a disease of late middle age.
2 Beriberi and pellagra are associated with depression.
3 Cycling between depression and mania accelerates with age.
4 Cushing's disease and thyroid disease are associated with depression.
5 In depressive psychosis, endocrine tests for Cushing's disease can be misleading.

Case 2
An impulsive act

History

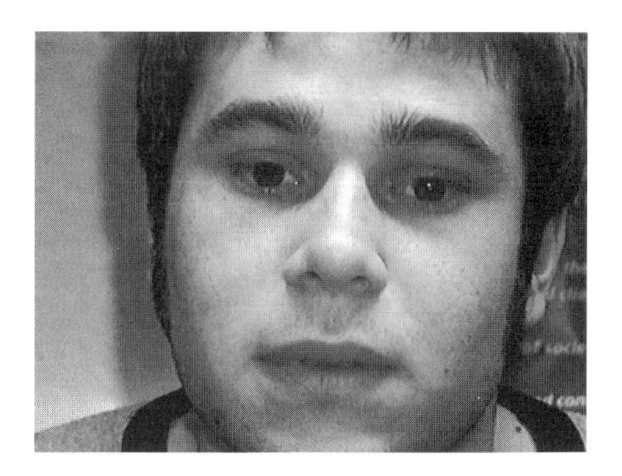

A 20-year-old student was seen in casualty following a deliberate but impulsive overdose of a combination of tablets. He was in the first term of the second year of his studies and had found in the weeks preceding his admission that he had been unable to concentrate on his work. This had led to increasing frustration and low mood which culminated in his taking an overdose. The decision to take the tablets was made on the spur of the moment and he regretted his action almost immediately. Nevertheless, on direct questioning, he did claim that he had wanted to end his life at that time. In retrospect, he did not think that the experience of taking the overdose, being admitted to hospital and being treated medically and psychiatrically had been useful.

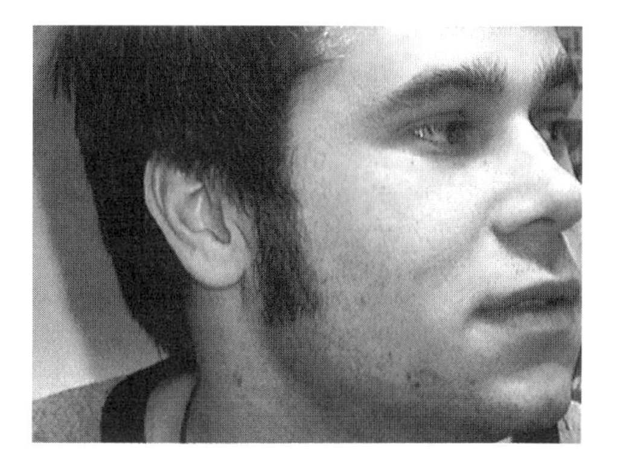

Notes

This very common but nevertheless dangerous and thought provoking incident is known as parasuicide. The patient had taken an overdose of paracetamol (acetominophen)* and aspirin.

A blood sample on admission, just over 4 h from the time of ingestion, before he was subjected to gastric lavage and dosed with a slurry of activated charcoal, showed an acetominophen level of 61 $mg\,L^{-1}$ and a salicylate level of 537 $mg\,L^{-1}$. The infusion of *N*-acetylcysteine, started soon after admission to hospital, was stopped. Five hours after admission, his salicylate level had dropped to 395 $mg\,L^{-1}$ and his acetominophen level was 34 $mg\,L^{-1}$.

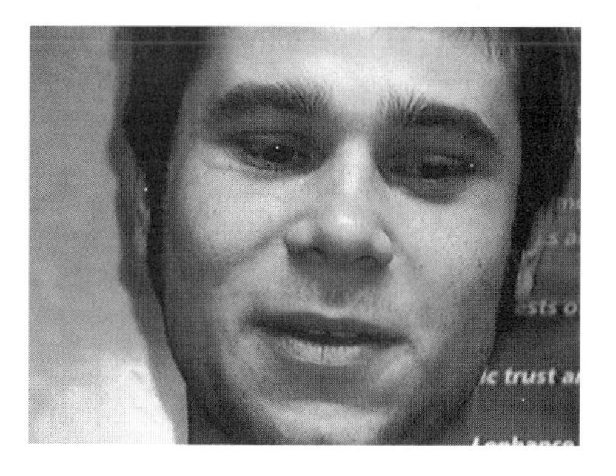

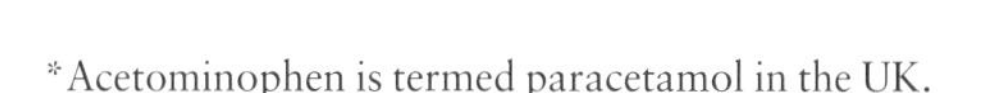

*Acetominophen is termed paracetamol in the UK.

Basic science

Acetominophen poisoning

The natural history of acetominophen poisoning is for non-specific signs, such as nausea, vomiting and lethargy, to be followed 24–48 h after ingestion by hepatocellular damage, manifesting as the elevation of serum transaminases, sometimes accompanied by tender hepatomegaly and jaundice and, in more severe poisoning, by acute liver failure with encephalopathy, bleeding and death.

Once the hepatic pathways of conjugation to sulphate or glucuronic acid are saturated, reactive metabolic intermediates of acetominophen become free to bind to liver macromolecules and cause necrosis. Treatment with a sulphydryl (S–H) donor, such as oral methionine, or an intravenous infusion of *N*-acetylcysteine, minimizes or prevents hepatocellular damage. If the patient presents after 4 h, a nomogram can be used to determine whether specific treatment is still warranted. Four hours after drug ingestion, an acetominophen level ≥200 mg L^{-1} warrants specific detoxifying treatment. Healthy patients with plasma acetominophen levels above this level have a 60% risk of sustaining serious liver damage if no treatment is given. Chronic alcoholics or patients taking enzyme-inducing drugs, such as phenytoin or carbamazepine, are at higher risk of acetominophen-induced hepatic necrosis and should be treated at an acetominophen level ≥100 mg L^{-1} at 4 h.

N-Acetylcysteine, which diverts the hepatotoxic effects of acetominophen by providing sulphydryl groups, has been shown to provide some protection up to 80 h after an acetominophen overdose. Provided that a donor organ can be found, liver transplantation, now accompanied by >60% survival, has transformed the prognosis of patients who go on to develop fulminant hepatic failure. The principal contraindications to liver transplantation are sepsis (which is implicated in 50% of deaths), haemodynamic instability and irreversible neurological damage.

Aspirin poisoning

The toxic dose of aspirin is very variable and symptoms correlate poorly with serum levels. Levels greater than 500 mg L^{-1} are usually associated with serious poisoning. Early symptoms include VIIIth nerve toxicity with reversible vertigo, tinnitus and impaired hearing. Respiratory alkalosis, due to excitation, and tachypnoea are followed by metabolic and respiratory acidosis, and impaired renal function through dehydration and hypotension.

Renal clearance of salicylate is greatly enhanced by maintaining urinary pH between 7 and 8. Intravenous treatment with bicarbonate and potassium ion replacement is used to maximize renal clearance of salicylate. Forced diuresis adds little to salicylate clearance over and above alkalinization of the urine. The latter is so effective that peritoneal dialysis or haemodialysis is rarely required.

Acute liver failure

In this patient, the initiation of treatment soon after ingestion of acetominophen and aspirin, together with subsequent evidence that the total absorbed dose had in any case been low, made the risk of liver damage remote. Even if the desire to die is fleeting, such an uncomplicated outcome is unfortunately not always the case. In acute liver failure, encephalopathy develops 8–28 days after the onset of jaundice. Patients have a marked prolongation of the prothrombin time, a high incidence of cerebral oedema and a high mortality. The mainstay of treatment of cerebral oedema is intravenous mannitol with prophylactic phenytoin to reduce the chance of occult seizure activity.

In subacute liver failure, the interval between the onset of jaundice and the development of encephalopathy is 4–12 weeks. Although the mortality is high, the disturbance of the prothrombin time is much less severe and the incidence of cerebral oedema is low. Indications for referral to a specialist centre are renal failure, typically with a creatinine level of over 200 μmol L^{-1}, and oliguria, encephalopathy and a prothrombin time of over 30 s.

Anxiety neuroses

For the individual concerned, parasuicide is far from a frivolous gesture. Although specific medical treatment to minimize organ damage often seems more productive than considering the underlying mental state of the patient, some understanding of the psychology of the neuroses is very useful.

The neuroses are a group of relatively common mental disorders in which the effects of common feelings and emotions are quantitatively rather than qualitatively abnormal. For example, a level of anxiety that prompts adequate preparation for a public speech or an examination (adaptive anxiety) is normal and may indeed be desirable. If the same situation produces anxiety that is so great as to be incapacitating, it falls into the category of anxiety neuroses. In an anxiety neurosis, feelings of dread, irritability or preoccupation, often accompanied by palpitations, sweating, breathlessness, tremor and insomnia, are disabling.

Panic disorder, which affects 1–2% of the population, is characterized by sudden, unexpected and overwhelming feelings of apprehension and terror that usually subside within 20 or 30 min. The condition has a genetic and familial component, and is most frequently observed in patients between late teenage and early twenties with a 2 : 1 female to male preponderance. Typical symptoms are flushing, sweating, light-headedness, palpitations, terror, dyspnoea, choking and feelings of impending doom, giving way to fatigue or exhaustion after the attack. The condition can lead to anxiety, attempts to avoid situations that the patient believes will induce an attack, drug or alcohol dependency, or depression. The differential diagnoses include:

- hyperthyroidism,
- phaeochromocytoma,
- complex partial seizures,
- hypoglycaemia, and
- alcohol or drug withdrawal.

Generalized anxiety disorder, unlike the tendency to panic attacks, is not genetic or familial. It is characterized by persistent anxiety that fluctuates little in intensity over a period of at least 1 month and often much longer. Symptoms of trembling, inability to relax, autonomic hyperactivity, anxiety, fear, insomnia and distractability are typical, and are sometimes compounded by alcohol or anxiolytic medication abuse.

Note: the suicide note shown on the CD was written by another patient (who survived).

MCQs

1 In acute liver failure, encephalopathy usually develops within 7 days.
2 *N*-Acetylcysteine decreases the metabolism of acetominophen to toxic intermediates.
3 Acetominophen itself is non-toxic.
4 Acute tubular necrosis is a complication of acetominophen poisoning.
5 Psychiatric intervention has a profound effect on life outcome in parasuicide.

Case 3
Breathlessness after a hysterectomy

History

A 44-year-old housewife and shop assistant was seen in accident and emergency with a 3-day history of worsening shortness of breath 2 weeks after an uneventful hysterectomy for uterine fibroids. She had been completely well until 10 days after the surgery when she woke up mildly short of breath with right-sided chest discomfort exacerbated by deep inspiration. Her husband prompted her to mention the problem to her doctor when he called around routinely to see how she was progressing after gynaecological surgery.

On examination, her blood pressure was 148/100 mmHg with a regular pulse of 120 beats per minute (b.p.m.). Examination of her respiratory system was completely normal apart from mild tachypnoea (20 min^{-1}). D dimer levels were 1.1 $mg L^{-1}$ (normal range $\leq$0.5 $mg L^{-1}$) and an isotope **ventilation/ perfusion scan** showed mismatched defects. An electrocardiogram (ECG) was normal apart from sinus tachycardia. Specifically, there were no signs of right heart strain or the 'S1, Q3, T3' pattern associated with pulmonary embolism.

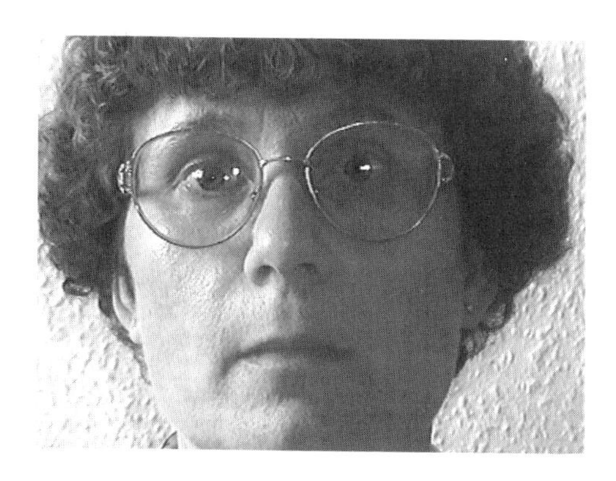

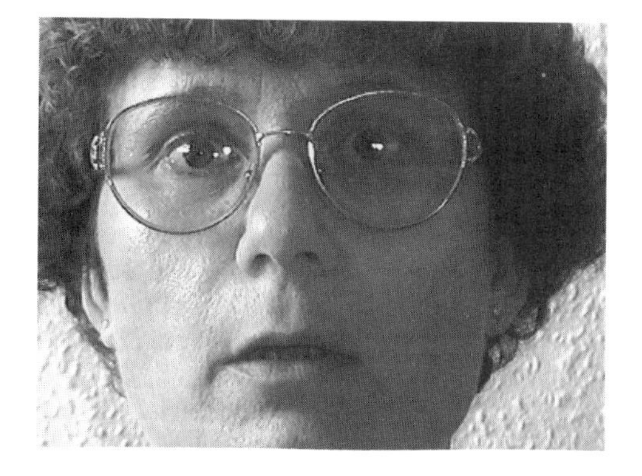

Notes

The patient had a deep venous thrombosis (DVT) in the thigh complicated by a pulmonary embolism.

The incidence of overt, spontaneous DVT increases from 0.2% between the ages of 65 and 69 years to 0.4% between 85 and 89 years. Signs such as pain, tenderness and swelling in the leg are non-specific and the diagnosis is often missed. Autopsy studies, however, show that venous thromboembolism accounts for no fewer than 10% of all hospital deaths.

High risk patients are those who have fractures or orthopaedic surgery to the lower limbs, hips or pelvis, major pelvic or abdominal surgery for cancer or trauma, patients with a previous history of DVT of pulmonary embolism, or those with lower limb paralysis or amputation.

The scenario in this case was particularly clear, but this diagnosis, which is one of the most frequent seen in hospital medicine, is fraught with difficulty. The associated chest pain suggests that the showers of emboli were small enough to reach the periphery of the lung and irritate the pleura. Larger pulmonary

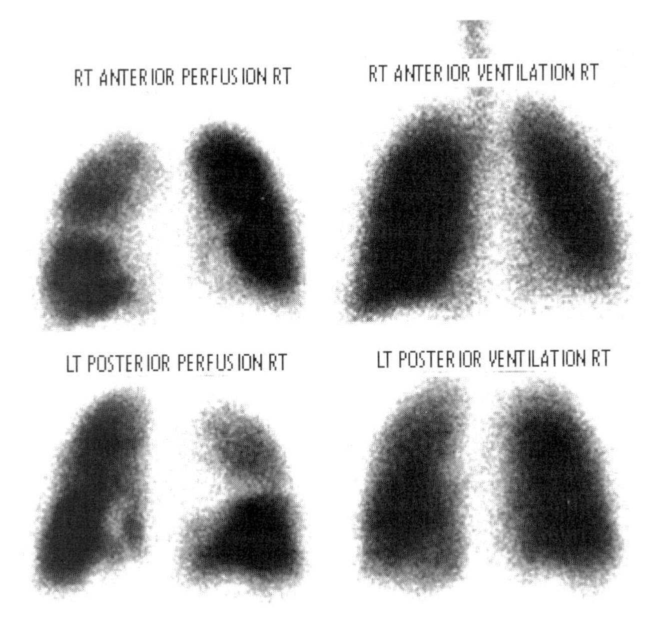

emboli block more central pulmonary arteries and present with breathlessness, sometimes associated with evidence of right heart strain on the ECG (right ventricular hypertrophy, right bundle branch block, ischaemic changes, an S wave in standard lead I and a Q wave and T wave flattening or inversion in standard lead III).

The action of the **fibrinolytic system** on intravascular blood clots produces a number of breakdown products including D dimers. A raised level of D dimers suggests an increase in intravascular coagulation, but is relatively non-specific. A normal circulating D dimer level ($\leq 0.5\,\mathrm{mg\,L^{-1}}$), in contrast, is said to be useful in excluding the presence of DVTs in 95% of cases.

In venography, contrast is injected into the small veins of the foot to outline the deep venous return in the leg. Flow artefacts, known as streaming, can produce a false positive result, and the test itself is associated with a small but significant risk of induction of a DVT. The test can also be uncomfortable for the patient, but is nevertheless the gold standard for DVT diagnosis.

Doppler studies are used to identify abnormal or absent flow in the deep veins of the leg. The test is highly specific and sensitive, but requires 20–30 min of an experienced radiologist's time.

The radioisotope ventilation/perfusion scan works by comparing the lung images produced by inhaling isotope with the images produced when isotope is injected intravenously. A matched deficit implies absence of air entry and perfusion typical of collapse, consolidation or other lung disease. A deficit in the perfusion scan with a normal ventilation scan indicates that normally ventilated lung is not being perfused and increases the probability that a pulmonary embolus is present. The sensitivity and specificity of this investigation are not as good as the widespread use of the procedure might suggest.

The definitive test to identify pulmonary emboli is a pulmonary angiogram. The test requires right heart catheterization, but is probably underused.

Basic science

Anticoagulants

Heparin, originally isolated from canine liver and from leeches, is a naturally occurring mucopolysaccharide polymer that binds to and greatly potentiates the activity of antithrombin III. It is an extremely potent anticoagulant that can dramatically reduce fibrin formation and thrombin generation. It is given either as a continual infusion or as subcutaneous or intravenous boluses to increase the partial thromboplastin time to twice the normal value. It is used for anticoagulation in pregnancy as coumarins are teratogenic, but is associated with rapid bone mineral loss and osteoporosis.

The major complication of heparin is bleeding. Although its effects can be rapidly reversed by protamine sulphate, its short half-life means that, in most cases, the use of specific antagonists is not necessary.

Low molecular weight heparins have long half-lives, so that single subcutaneous doses produce 24-h anticoagulant cover by inactivating activated factor X. As doses adjusted on the basis of body weight have predictable anticoagulant activity, laboratory monitoring or prolonged inpatient stays are unnecessary. Intravenous heparin is still the treatment of choice for pulmonary embolism.

Warfarin is a coumarin that acts by inhibiting the normal decarboxylation of newly produced vitamin K-dependent clotting factors II, VII, IX and X. The effects of warfarin are specifically antagonized by vitamin K. The dose is adjusted and balanced so that the International Normalized Ratio (INR) is 1.4 or greater. An increase in warfarin dose or a reduction in the ability of the liver to synthesize proteins (such as the onset of mild heart failure—a much more potent cause of warfarin-associated bleeding than is the concurrent ingestion of drugs such as antibiotics) results in over-anticoagulation.

Factors that predispose to deep venous thrombosis

- Bed rest
- Old age and immobility
- Clotting diathesis, e.g. inherited deficiency of protein C or protein S
- Hyperosmolar coma
- Surgery, particularly orthopaedic surgery of the hip and knee
- Previous deep vein thrombosis
- Lupus anticoagulant
- Malignancy
- Paroxysmal nocturnal haemoglobinuria
- Behçet's syndrome
- Trauma
- Obesity

Inherited thrombophilias

Less well known than the coagulation defects such as haemophilia (factor VIII deficiency), the molecular mechanisms behind the inherited thrombophilias are only just being elucidated. A relevant prothrombotic factor can now be identified in ≈ 50% of patients presenting with venous thrombosis.

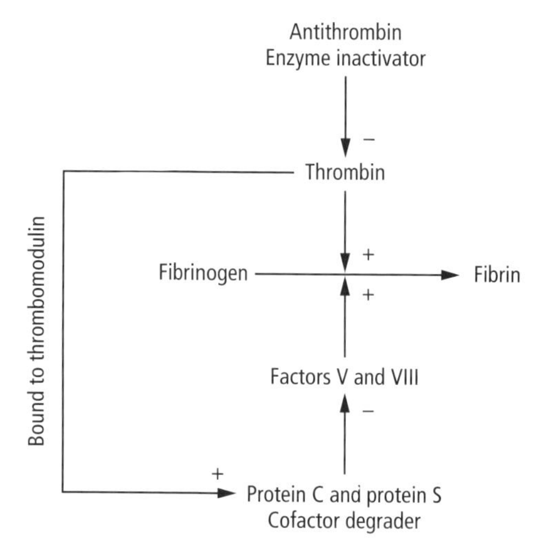

High plasma levels of homocysteine in homocystinuria predispose to thrombosis. There is some evidence that more modestly raised levels (present in 20% of those with thrombosis) have a similar effect. Mutations of the genes encoding antithrombin, protein C and protein S are implicated in inherited thrombophilias. The annual risk of thrombosis in a heterozygous protein C or S deficiency is 2% (i.e. 20–30 times normal). Approximately 10% of patients who present with their first DVT have a defect in one of these. The homozygous state is usually lethal at birth. High plasma levels of factor VIII are present in 20–25% of patients who present with a venous thrombosis. A causal association seems likely, but has not been proven as yet. Factor V Leiden, a mutation of factor V that renders it resistant to the effects of protein C, has a gene frequency of 5–10% in Europe, but is very rare in Japanese and Africans. The annual risk of thrombosis in a heterozygote is 1%, and about 8% in a homozygote.

MCQs

1 The absence of ECG changes excludes significant pulmonary embolism.
2 Heparin acts by binding to and inactivating antithrombin III.
3 Warfarin acts by impairing the production of vitamin K-dependent clotting factors.
4 Pulmonary angiography is the gold standard for the diagnosis of pulmonary emboli.
5 In the absence of signs in the legs, pulmonary embolus is a rare cause of sudden breathlessness.

Case 4
The jeans that wouldn't do up

History

A 56-year-old counsellor for alcoholics was seen in clinic with a 5-year history of depression and low mood. She had received many reassurances about her condition that had at various times been ascribed to a degree of social isolation, lack of direction, postviral fatigue syndrome and stress. At one time, many years previously, a jejunal biopsy had shown unequivocal coeliac disease, but the villous atrophy did not appear to be modified by a gluten-free diet and she was lost to follow-up. Other past medical problems were thyrotoxicosis, sciatica and endometriosis.

While standing at the mirror, she noticed a lower abdominal swelling that prevented her from doing her jeans up, and duly presented to her GP who palpated the mass bimanually, made a provisional diagnosis of a fibroid uterus and, after some persuasion, referred her to the local gynaecology clinic. While waiting for an appointment to be sent, the patient noticed that she was being woken by breathlessness at night and assumed that her childhood asthma had returned. She returned to her GP and was sent with some urgency to the gynaecologist who carried out a laparotomy.

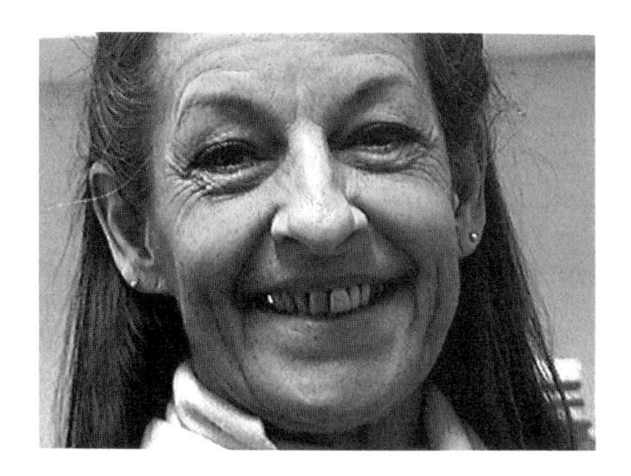

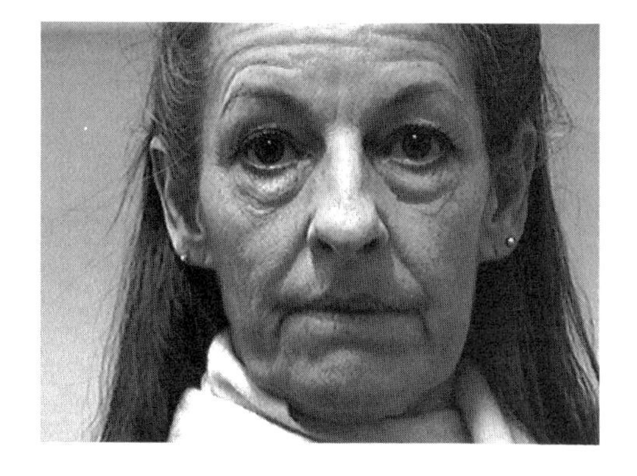

Notes

The patient was found to have ovarian cancer presenting with ascites and a pleural effusion.

The ultrasound examination showed the uterus to be normal in shape, size and echotexture. There was an 11.5-cm × 9.5-cm × 9-cm cystic mass arising out of the pelvis with a single loculation within it. A large, right **pleural effusion** was noted. At surgery, secondary deposits were seen to be studded throughout her omentum and peritoneum, together with a small amount of ascites. A large ovarian tumour was biopsied.

Ovarian cancer is the fourth most common cause of cancer death in women. Although survival is very good in early disease, as symptoms and signs are often absent until the disease is extensive, the overall outcome of the condition is poor. Most ovarian tumours are derived from the epithelial component of the ovaries, but the stromal cells, germ cells and, rarely, the mesenchymal cells can also be implicated. The tumour stage, the presence of ascites, the age of the patient, the histological type and grade, as well as the cellular deoxyribonucleic acid (DNA) content and mitotic activity index, are of prognostic value in these tumours.

Stromal cell tumours account for 10% of ovarian tumours and are largely responsible for the hormone-secreting subtypes. Excessive oestrogen production produces precocious puberty in childhood or dysfunctional bleeding in postmenopausal women. During reproductive life, the detection of excess oestrogen production is more challenging as menstrual irregularities develop insidiously. Excessive androgen production, leading to hirsutism and virilism (change in body habitus, deepening of the voice and clitoromegaly), is often more obvious. Germ cell tumours can produce α-fetoprotein or excessive human chorionic gonadotrophin (hCG), producing a feminizing syndrome or even hyperthyroidism. Most, however, are epithelial and the non-specific symptoms of increasing abdominal girth, abdominal discomfort and menstrual irregularity are often ignored until it is too late.

Basic science

Ascites

Ascites, the presence of free fluid in the peritoneal cavity, is most commonly associated with intra-abdominal malignancies and portal hypertension resulting from alcohol-induced hepatic cirrhosis. In cirrhosis, the primary causative event in the formation of ascites—whether vascular underfilling leading to renal compensation or primary retention of salt and water—is unclear. Ascites is infrequent in cirrhosis unless portal hypertension, which raises hydrostatic pressure within the splanchnic capillary bed, and hypoalbuminaemia, which reduces plasma oncotic pressure, are also present. Hepatic lymph may also weep into the peritoneal cavity.

Other causes of ascites can be deduced logically by considering conditions that either reduce intravascular osmotic pressure or increase portal blood pressure. Examples of the former are poor protein intake, for example kwashiorkor, or excessive protein loss, such as the nephrotic syndrome or protein-losing enteropathy. Portal pressure can be increased by portal vein thrombosis, compression of the portal vein by tumour or lymphadenopathy, hepatic vein thrombosis (Budd–Chiari syndrome), obstruction of the inferior vena cava by thromboembolic disease or compression, or increased right heart pressure, for example congestive cardiac failure or, rarely, constrictive pericarditis. Tuberculous peritonitis is a rare cause of ascites, but should be considered in patients from the Asian subcontinent.

Accumulation of fluid in the abdominal

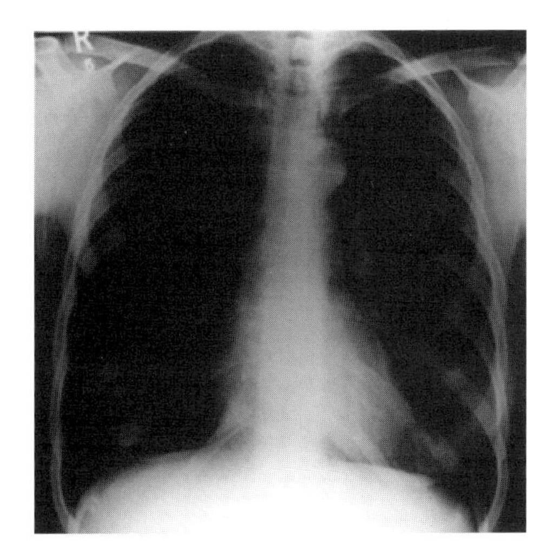

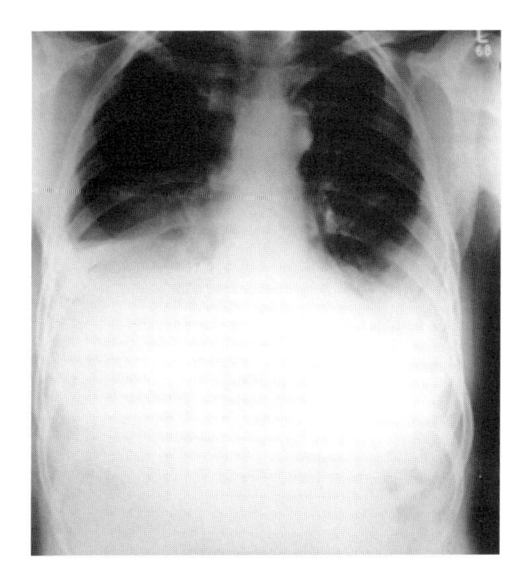

cavity is usually painless unless pancreatitis, hepatoma or peritonitis is present. Direct pressure from tense ascites can cause indigestion and heartburn, and diaphragmatic splinting and associated pleural effusions (more often on the right) lead to dyspnoea and orthopnoea (as was the case here).

In uncomplicated cirrhosis (as well as congestive cardiac failure and nephrotic syndrome), ascitic fluid has the characteristics of a transudate rather than an exudate. The fluid is straw coloured, has no blood staining, fewer than 250 white blood cells mm^{-3} and less than 30 g protein L^{-1}.

Ovarian function

The ovaries produce oestradiol from the granulosa cells that form the developing follicles, androgens from the theca cells that surround them (most of which is aromatized to oestrogens by the granulosa cells) and progesterone from the corpora lutea that develop after ovulation. The corpus luteum is a temporary endocrine organ that secretes progesterone to prepare the oestradiol-primed endometrium to accept the newly fertilized ovum and to facilitate the establishment of early pregnancy.

Ovarian development

In the presence of two complete X chromosomes, the wolffian ducts regress and the müllerian ducts form the fallopian tubes, uterus and upper part of the vagina. The ovaries develop to contain granulosa cells, stromal cells and ova. As formation of the fallopian tubes, the uterus and the upper third of the vagina from the müllerian ducts is entirely independent of ovarian development, these structures are almost normal in conditions in which the ovaries fail to develop, such as Turner's syndrome (45 XO genotype). The phenotypic sex, the external genitalia, however, is dependent on the type of gonad formed, and the type of gonad depends on the presence or absence of the sex-determining region of the Y chromosome. In the female, the genital tubercle becomes the clitoris, the genital swellings either side, the labia majora and the urethral fold, the labia minora.

Symptoms, signs and tests used to define ovarian function

The vagina and endometrium, bone and breasts are all major oestrogen target tissues. Prolonged absence of oestrogen during pubertal development will impair breast development, and oestrogen deprivation at other times predisposes to bone mineral loss and cardiovascular disease. More immediate markers of oestrogen activity are endometrial proliferation and vaginal lubrication. Absence of oestrogens leads to dyspareunia—painful sexual intercourse—and persistently low oestrogen levels produce amenorrhoea. Amenorrhoea can also occur in the presence of oestrogen.

An elevated blood progesterone level measured between days 19 and 21 of the menstrual cycle is a very simple and useful indicator of the presence of a corpus luteum, which itself is an indicator that ovulation must have occurred.

Transvaginal ultrasound or magnetic resonance imaging is useful to demonstrate streak ovaries, ovarian tumours, polycystic ovaries and the presence and size of follicles during ovulation induction.

MCQs

1 Most ovarian cancers are non-hormone secreting.
2 The secreting subtypes of ovarian cancer are usually derived from epithelial cells.
3 Development of the fallopian tubes and uterus depends on the presence of normal ovaries.
4 The theca cells of the ovary produce androgens.
5 Pain on sexual intercourse is a symptom of progesterone withdrawal.

Case 5
Headache, falls and weakness

History

A 78-year-old retired odd job man and lorry driver was admitted to hospital with a 6-day history of right-sided weakness, headaches and falls. He claimed that his right arm 'went dead' 6 days previously and that, on the morning of admission to hospital, his right leg had become 'numb' and he had found it difficult to 'get his words out'. Neither he nor his wife thought it appropriate to take action until he fell over and bruised his right arm while attempting to stand up after opening his bowels. Since the development of weakness in his arm, he had also been aware of headaches. These had not particularly disturbed him, however, and they were certainly less intense than the migraine headaches he used to get during his 4 years as a prisoner of war in the Far East.

Examination was demanding as the patient found it difficult to cooperate. His blood pressure was 168/82 mmHg supine with a pulse of 84 beats per minute. His sublingual temperature was 38.4 °C, and he was noted to have reduced power and mildly increased tone in the right arm and leg. Tendon reflexes were increased on that side and both plantar responses were upgoing. Fundoscopy was normal. Approximately 2 h after admission he had a *grand mal* convulsion and, 15 min later, a further fit without fully recovering from the first. Re-examination at that time revealed mild neck stiffness.

A computed tomography (CT) scan to exclude raised intracranial pressure was followed by a lumbar puncture, which showed increased protein (1.8 g L^{-1}) and 8000 white cells mm^{-3} with a low glucose level. Gram-negative cocci were seen on microscopy of the cerebrospinal fluid (CSF), and were subsequently grown from his blood.

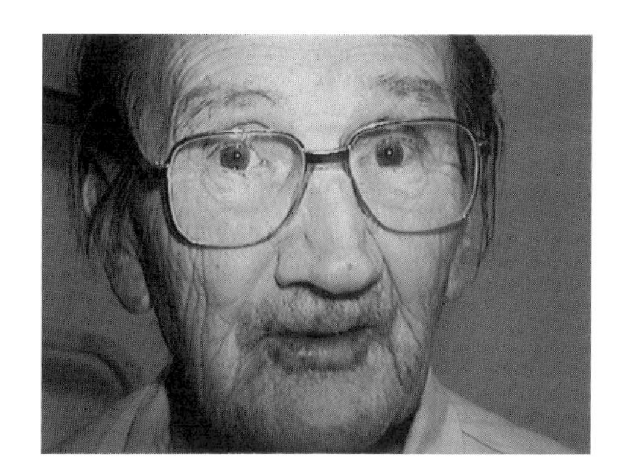

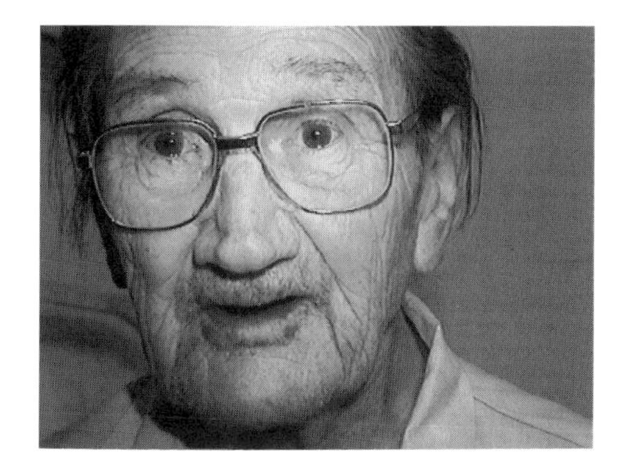

Notes

The patient was suffering from meningococcal meningitis.

The effects of inflammation in the subarachnoid space are severe headache, fever, drowsiness, vomiting and reduced conscious level which, untreated, rapidly lead to convulsions and coma. Neck stiffness—involuntary resistance to passive movement—is the classical physical sign of meningitis. Kernig's sign, pain and muscle spasm, induced by flexing the thigh with the knee extended or by extending the flexed knee with the thigh flexed, is another commonly used test of meningeal irritation.

In 25% of patients, meningitis develops very rapidly and patients become seriously ill or die with marked cerebral oedema within 24 h of the start of symptomatology. In 50%, meningitis develops over 1–7 days in association with respiratory symptoms and, in a further 20%, meningitis develops over an even longer time course following 1–3 weeks of respiratory symptoms.

Basic science

Bacterial meningitis can result from the spread of infectious organisms to the pia-arachnoid from adjacent structures, such as the paranasal sinuses, following cranial penetration, such as trauma or neurosurgery, or more usually as a result of haematogenous spread. As there are no barriers to the rapid spread of infectious organisms within the CSF space, inflammation invariably extends throughout the pia-arachnoid—surrounding the spinal cord, brain, cerebral ventricles, choroid plexus and cranial nerves including the optic nerve. The inflammation of the pia-arachnoid leads to the accumulation of pus in the CSF which may cause hydrocephalus by interfering with CSF flow. The infective agent and the toxins it produces may also damage the central nervous system directly.

Table 5.1 Infective causes of meningitis

Organism	Clinical features	Cerebrospinal fluid
Meningococcus Gram-negative diplococci 20% of adult and 30% of childhood meningitis	Purpuric rash Septicaemic shock	Neutrophils 500–2000 mm^{-3} Protein 1–3 $g\,L^{-1}$ Glucose very low
Pneumococcus Gram-positive diplococci 40% of adult and 15% of childhood meningitis	Cranial nerve damage Otitis media Lobar pneumonia High mortality (10–20%)	Neutrophils 500–2000 mm^{-3} Protein 1–3 $g\,L^{-1}$ Glucose very low
Haemophilus influenzae Gram-negative bacilli 50% of childhood and 2% of adult meningitis	Commonest in children under 5 years	Neutrophils 500–2000 mm^{-3} Protein 1–3 $g\,L^{-1}$ Glucose very low
Coxsackie virus and echovirus. Rising antibody titre and positive throat swab		Lymphocytes 50–500 mm^{-3} Protein 0.5–1 $g\,L^{-1}$ Glucose normal
Mumps Rising antibody titre and positive throat swab		Lymphocytes 50–500 mm^{-3} Protein 0.5–1 $g\,L^{-1}$ Glucose normal
Mycobacterium tuberculosis Acid- and alcohol-fast bacilli Ziehl–Nielsen staining	Subacute onset Cranial nerve lesions Fits in children Pyrexia of unknown origin	Lymphocytes 100–600 mm^{-3} Protein 1–6 $g\,L^{-1}$ Glucose low ($<1.4\,mmol\,L^{-1}$)
Leptospira icterohaemorrhagica (Weil's disease) Rising serum antibody titre	Following exposure to rat urine Associated with hepatitis and nephritis. A high peripheral white cell count is typical	Lymphocytes 200–300 mm^{-3} Protein 0.5–1.5 $g\,L^{-1}$ Glucose normal

Streptococcus pneumoniae and *Neisseria meningitidis* (meningococcus) are responsible for most cases of bacterial meningitis in adults. In children, *Haemophilus influenzae* type B is also an important cause of meningitis. In people over the age of 50 years, almost 20% of cases of bacterial meningitis are caused by Gram-negative enteric bacteria.

Meningococcal meningitis is often responsible for epidemics of meningitis, and very rapidly evolving disease associated with a purpuric, ecchymotic, petechial or sometimes measles-like skin rash (in around 50% of cases) should suggest the diagnosis and lead to antibiotic treatment as a medical emergency.

MCQs

1 Untreated, 90% of cases of meningococcal meningitis lead to death within 24 h.
2 Neck stiffness in meningitis is caused by the hydraulic effects of increased CSF pressure.
3 The usual causative organisms in adults are meningococcus and *Haemophilus*.
4 Infection and inflammation in meningitis usually spare the distal spinal cord.
5 The main threat of meningitis is spread of infection to the brain tissue itself.

Case 6
Swelling of tongue and face

History

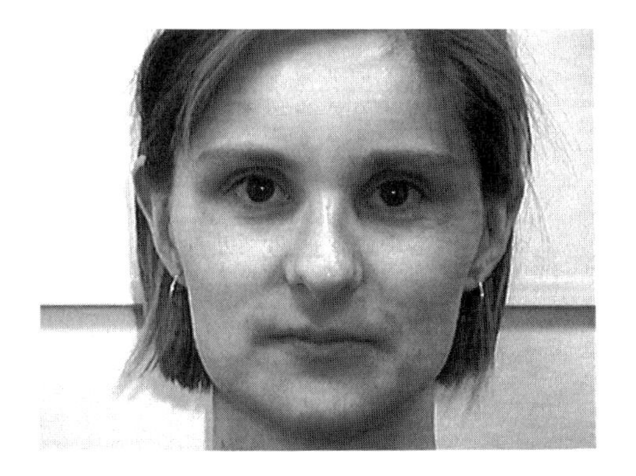

A 27-year-old housewife was admitted to hospital with a short history of swelling on her face and in her mouth and throat. She had noticed a single painless lump on her chin the day before admission, and assumed that she was going to develop 'a huge spot'. Later the same day, however, a number of similar painless swellings appeared on her face, and she was woken at 4 a.m. the following morning by breathlessness. The swelling had extended to her forehead and limbs, and she realized that swelling of her pharynx and tongue was obstructing her breathing. An ambulance was called and she was admitted to hospital. She denied any previous history of infection, asthma, hay fever, eczema or allergic reactions of any kind, and had no specific family history of the same. She had not eaten any unusual foods or food that she had not eaten before, but had consumed a chocolate-coated peanut bar. A serum sample for mast cell tryptase (several hours after the presumed start of the reaction) was within normal limits.

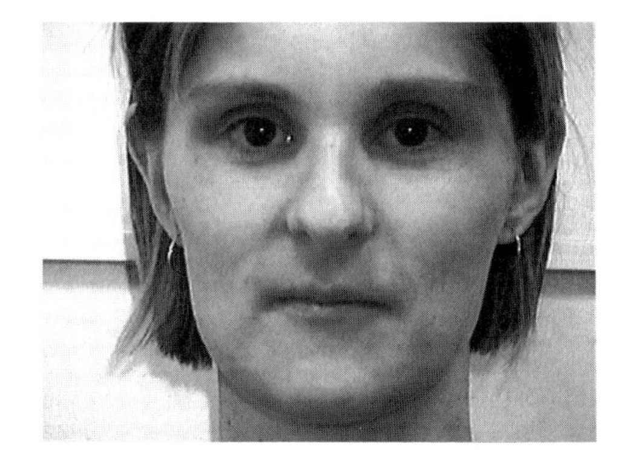

Notes

The patient had facial and laryngeal angio-oedema and was subsequently shown to be allergic to peanuts.

The tendency to make immunoglobulin E (IgE) antibodies to ingested antigens is inherited, but environmental factors are also important. Peanut allergy produces more severe symptoms than many other allergic reactions, and more than 10% of patients with the problem have had to be admitted to hospital at some time with symptoms that have required adrenaline (epinephrine) treatment, such as abdominal pain and collapse. Facial angio-oedema is the commonest

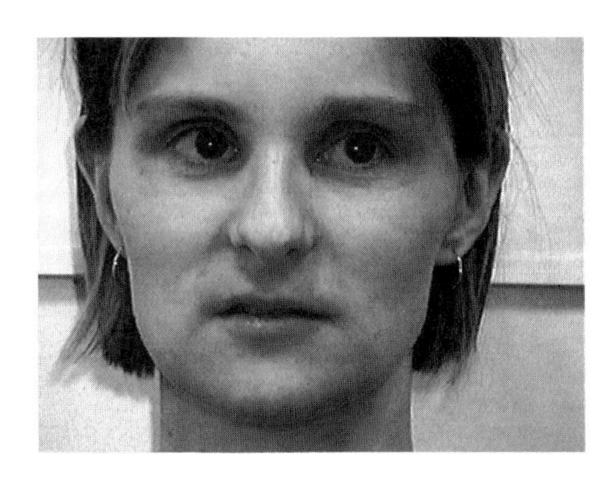

symptom (as was the case here). Other symptoms, such as hypotension, erythema, pruritus, urticaria, vomiting, abdominal pain, rhinitis and conjunctivitis, are variable. Chest pain, convulsions and incontinence are rare, and laryngeal oedema is the symptom that most commonly proves fatal if the condition remains untreated.

In most cases, peanut allergy manifests in childhood, and allergies to a variety of other antigens appear with age, together with symptoms of atopy, such as eczema, asthma and allergic rhinitis. Skin-prick testing and peanut-specific IgE levels do not predict the clinical severity of the condition and, because as little as 100 μg of peanut protein can elicit a response, contamination or minimal use of peanut products in prepared food can be a cause for concern.

Mast cell tryptase is usually raised about 1 h after an anaphylactic or anaphylactoid (i.e. mast cell degranulation, but not through an IgE-mediated immune mechanism) reaction. If elevated levels of IgE are found in patients suspected of having had an anaphylactic reaction, specific allergens can sometimes be identified using skin-prick tests or radioallergosorbent (RAST) testing.

Basic science

The definition of anaphylaxis is imprecise. Anaphylactic reactions are severe, systemic allergic reactions characterized either by hypotension or by the development of bronchospasm or laryngeal oedema. They are type I allergic reactions, mediated by specific IgE antibodies bound to specific high affinity receptors on the surface of mast cells and basophils. When cross-linked by antigen, the receptors induce the rapid release of chemical mediators of inflammation, such as histamine, and proteolytic enzymes, such as tryptase, proteoglycans, leukotrienes and prostaglandins. These cause rapid vasodilatation, increased capillary leakage, rashes, mucosal oedema and smooth muscle contraction (with abdominal pain or other symptoms), that develop within 5–10 min of exposure, and increase to a full-blown reaction usually within 10–30 min. Allergy to latex rubber, absorbed through the skin or across mucosal surfaces, is also relatively common, but produces reactions somewhat later (>30 min). Intravenous administration of antigen, such as a drug, most commonly causes hypotension and cardiovascular collapse with fainting. Ingested allergens more typically cause respiratory difficulty that can progress to asphyxia. Insect stings cause both of these reactions in equal proportions.

Emergency treatment consists of intramuscular epinephrine (0.5 mL of a 1 mg mL^{-1} (1/1000) solution), with a second dose after a few minutes if there is no improvement. This should be followed by antihistamines (10 mg of chlorpheniramine intramuscularly (i.m.) or intravenously (i.v.)) and hydrocortisone (200 mg i.m. or i.v.).

MCQs

1 Peanut allergy tends to produce severe allergic reactions.
2 The tendency to make IgE antibodies to ingested antigens is inherited.
3 Skin-prick testing and peanut-specific IgE levels predict the clinical severity of the condition.
4 Anaphylactic reactions are type I allergic reactions.
5 Anaphylactic reactions to injected drugs typically cause bronchospasm and asphyxia.

Case 7
Back and chest pain, headaches and haemoptysis

History

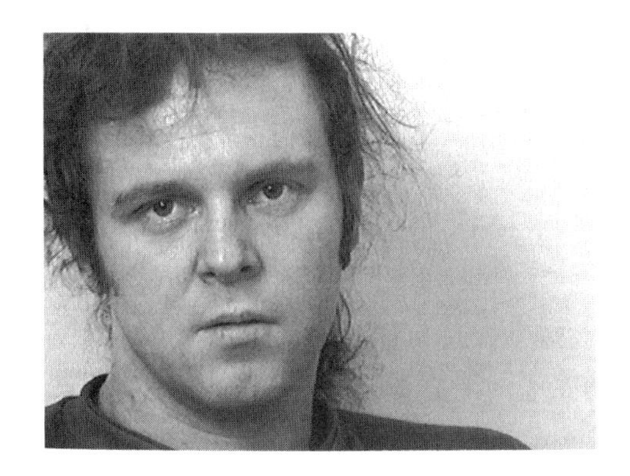

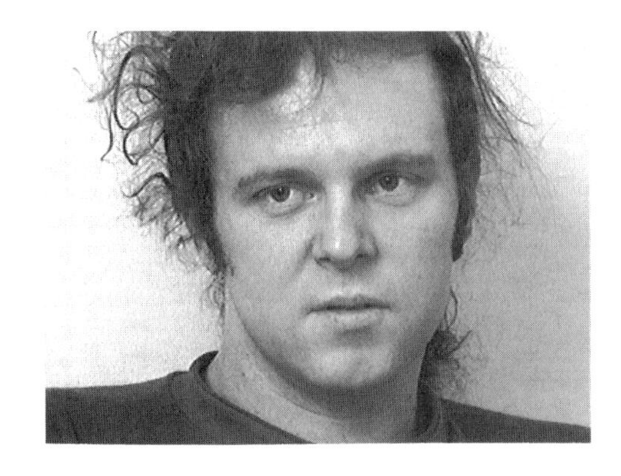

A 23-year-old student, who had previously been entirely well, was admitted through accident and emergency with a 2-day history of pain in his back and chest, headaches and haemoptysis. He had been 'sitting around at his friend's house' when he first began to feel sweaty, shivery and cold. He returned home and retired to bed with a temperature of 103 °F (39.4 °C). By the following morning, he had developed a frontal headache that was greatly exacerbated by coughing, and pain in the lower back which he took to be a muscle that he had 'pulled' through 'tensing up'. The next day he saw his doctor who diagnosed a virus infection, but, as the back pain, headaches and the deep, dull chest pain continued the following day and were accompanied by haemoptyses, he was referred to hospital.

On examination, he had a temperature of 38.2 °C and was anxious and uncomfortable. He was noted to have rapid, shallow breathing and was clearly in pain when coughing up a small amount of purulent, blood-stained sputum. Auscultation of his chest revealed right mid and lower zone crackles with bronchial breathing at the right base. A chest X-ray was requested.

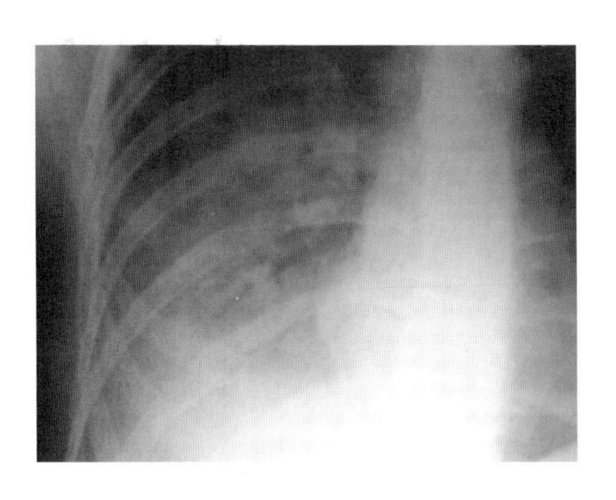

Notes

The patient had (pneumococcal) lobar pneumonia.

Pneumonia, inflammation of the lung parenchyma beyond the terminal bronchioles, may be caused by a number of different chemical, immune/allergic and microbial insults. In common usage, the term refers to the response to infective organisms reaching the lung through inhalation, aspiration from the

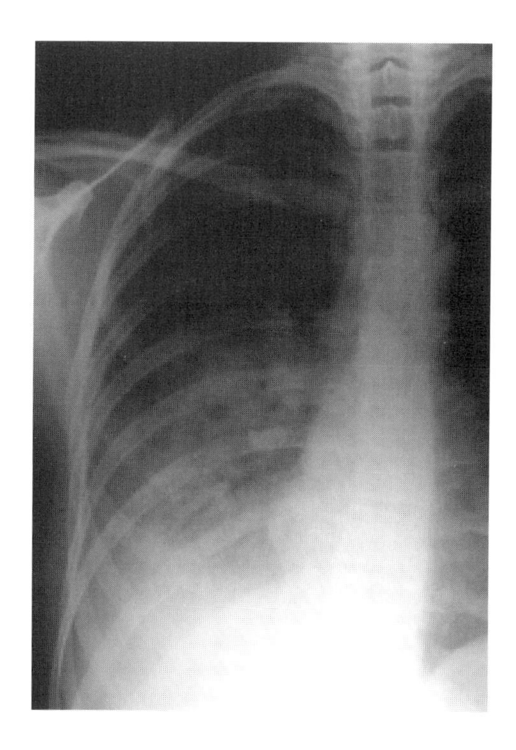

nasopharynx or oropharynx or, less usually, haematogenous spread from a distant site of infection or direct spread from an adjacent source of infection such as a penetrating injury or abscess. The presence of an organism in the sputum does not necessarily implicate it in the underlying disease.

As pneumonic consolidation progresses, gas exchange is progressively reduced, but, as perfusion of the affected area continues, an effective right to left shunt develops that decreases P_aO_2. Unaffected areas of the lung may be hyperventilated and P_aO_2 may be maintained, sometimes in association with a decrease in P_aCO_2. The compliance of the lung is decreased in pneumonia and, even in the absence of the constraints imposed by pleuritic pain, reduced tidal volume and increased respiratory rate become the most energy-effective pattern of breathing.

Typical viral causes of pneumonia are:

- respiratory syncytial virus in infants and
- parainfluenza, adenoviruses and rhinoviruses in adults,

either leading directly to a pneumonic reaction or allowing commensal flora to overgrow. Depending on the presence of pre-existing disease, the main bacterial and atypical causes are:

- *Streptococcus pneumoniae*,
- *Staphylococcus pyogenes*,
- *Klebsiella pneumoniae*,
- *Bordetella pertussis*,
- *Mycobacterium tuberculosis*,
- *Mycoplasma pneumoniae*,
- *Legionella* spp., and
- *Chlamydia pneumoniae*.

In immunosuppressed patients, *Pneumocystis carinii*, cytomegalovirus infections and atypical *Mycobacterium* infections are relatively common.

Basic science

Bronchial breathing

Bronchial breathing is one of the most useful and informative signs in clinical medicine. Under normal conditions, the sound of air moving in and out of the major airways is muffled by the surrounding layer of relatively static air in the alveoli, in exactly the same way that soft, foamy materials are used as ear defenders and as insulators to reduce transmitted sounds from machinery. If the sound-deadening alveolar 'foam' is filled with pus and debris (as occurs in pneumonic consolidation) or increased in rigidity (i.e. lung fibrosis), the insulating effect is lost, and the sound of air passing through the major airways is transmitted clearly to the periphery as so-called 'bronchial breathing'.

Gas exchange

External respiration is the absorption of oxygen and the excretion of carbon dioxide from the body. Internal respiration is the exchange of gas between cells and cell fluid. At rest, 12–15 breaths per minute move 6–8 L of air into and out of the airways. The air mixes with alveolar gas and, by simple diffusion through a fine layer of surfactant produced by type II pneumocytes and through an epithelium of type I pneumocytes and capillary endothelium separated by a basement membrane, 250 mL of oxygen enters red cells passing through pulmonary capillaries and 200 mL of carbon dioxide is excreted.

Normal airflow with each breath moves the 'tidal volume'. Of this, approximately 150 mL fills the anatomical 'dead space'—conducting airways between the mouth and respiratory bronchioles that have no gas exchange capability. At the end of a quiet expiration, the air remaining within the lungs is the 'functional residual capacity', a proportion of which can be exhaled by a conscious exhalatory effort. The air that remains in the lung after a full expiratory effort is the margin that makes the 'total lung capacity' bigger than the 'vital capacity', which is the maximum volume that can be exhaled after a full inspiratory effort.

Antibiotic resistance

In the UK, the incidence of community-acquired pneumonia is between 1 and 5 per 1000 per year, broadly matching the levels in France, Holland and Canada. There is increasing and justified concern that, after over 50 years of effective control, the indiscriminate use of antibiotics has led to the re-emergence of tuberculosis, typhoid fever, meningitis, pneumonia and septicaemias as global threats. In addition to the now well-established antibiotic resistance of *Haemophilus influenzae* and a number of other Gram-negative bacilli, *Streptococcus pneumoniae*, one of the most prevalent pathogens in community-acquired pneumonia, has also shown signs of resistance. The consensus guidelines produced by the British Thoracic Society, the American Thoracic Society and Expert Panels in Canada and France emphasize different management depending on the severity of the condition and whether the setting is hospital or community based. Currently, mild or moderate pneumococcal pneumonia is still thought likely to respond to a sufficient dose of amoxycillin or penicillin G. In severe infection, initial therapy should be broad spectrum and promptly administered.

MCQs

1 Bronchial breathing is heard in pulmonary fibrosis and pneumothorax.
2 In health, the anatomical dead space in adulthood is typically 250 mL.
3 In consolidated lung, a left to right shunt can cause arterial oxygen desaturation.
4 Rapid, deep breathing is characteristically seen in patients with pneumonia.
5 Surfactant is produced by type II pneumocytes.

Case 8
A cough and a rash

History

A 45-year-old taxi driver, who had previously been completely well apart from a mild upper respiratory tract infection some weeks earlier, woke one morning to find a rash on his back, arms and palate. It was dark, purplish red and punctate, although in places the lesions were so close together that they appeared to produce an almost confluent rash. As it was painless and not irritating he did not take much notice of it, but did observe that when he brushed his teeth his gums would bleed more easily than normal. Although the rash spread onto his limbs during the next 3 days, he continued to dismiss it until his girlfriend, who had been reading about the association of a rash with meningitis, became anxious and insisted that he seek help. His doctor took a blood sample and explained that the result would take a few days to come back. Having decided to take a day off work, he went home and was surprised to receive a telephone call from the hospital that same afternoon asking him to attend casualty.

He had been involved in a road traffic accident in the previous year in which he sustained minor injuries. His only medication during the previous 6 months was occasional ibuprofen for headaches.

On examination, he was noted to have a dense, petechial rash on his trunk, limbs and fauces, with a large ecchymosis on his right arm. There was no lymphadenopathy and no hepatomegaly or splenomegaly. The full blood count that elicited the telephone call was normal apart from a platelet count of $10 \times 10^{9}\,L^{-1}$ (normal range = 150–400 $\times 10^{9}\,L^{-1}$). A repeat platelet count showed a level of $16 \times 10^{9}\,L^{-1}$.

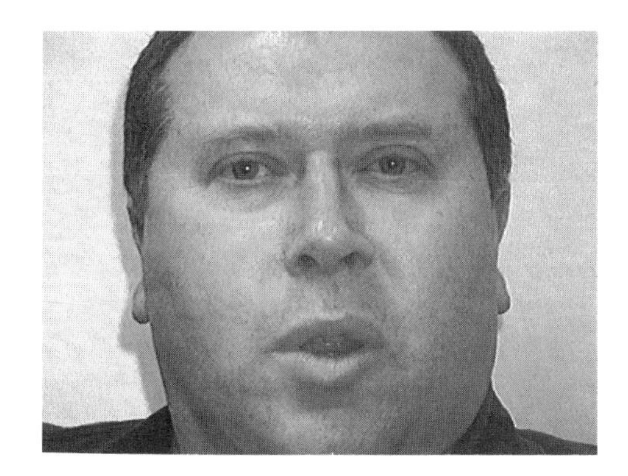

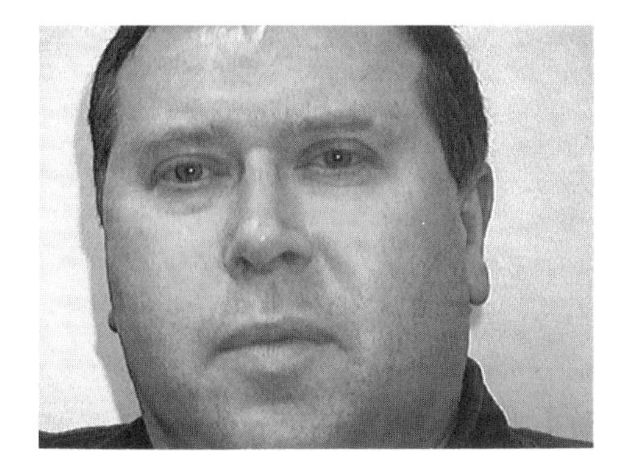

Notes

The patient had developed idiopathic thrombocytopenic purpura as a complication of a viral chest infection 3 weeks previously. On treatment with high dose glucocorticoids, the rash very slowly began to improve and the platelet count increased to within normal limits. The patient noted very prominent glucocorticoid side-effects of appetite stimulation, and both he and his girlfriend complained bitterly about his mood swings.

Thrombocytopenia is caused by:

- decreased platelet production,
- increased platelet destruction or
- sequestration of platelets by the spleen.

In idiopathic thrombocytopenic purpura, as was the case here, the principal problem was excessive, immune-mediated destruction of circulating platelets. In children, sudden thrombocytopenia in the recovery phase after an upper respiratory tract infection accounts for 90% of cases. Few patients develop serious complications or long-term sequelae and, as most of them recover completely within 6 months, few require specific treatment. Transient immune thrombocytopenia can also complicate infectious mononucleosis, viral hepatitis and other viral illnesses, and sudden thrombocytopenia can also be an unusual presenting feature of metastatic tumour, aplastic anaemia and acute leukaemia, or can occur in systemic lupus erythematosus.

The two mechanisms that are thought to cause platelet destruction in idiopathic thrombocytopenic purpura are the production of antiviral antibodies against glycoprotein antigens that cross-react with platelet antigens, or platelet (Fc) antibody receptor binding by immune complexes containing viral antigens. Megakaryocytes in the bone marrow are usually normal or increased in number. The risk of intracranial and other bleeds is substantial when platelet counts fall to less than $20 \times 10^9\,L^{-1}$.

Basic science

Platelet production

Platelets are small, granulated bodies between 2 and 4 μm in diameter. They are produced by the fragmentation of megakaryocytes, which are very large bone marrow cells that have undergone several cycles of DNA replication without cell division, making them strikingly polyploid. Around one-third of all platelets produced are sequestered by the spleen, but the remainder circulate for 7–10 days, become senescent and are removed from the circulation. Platelet numbers are maintained between about 150×10^9 and $400 \times 10^9\,L^{-1}$, but can increase rapidly in systemic inflammation, tumours, haemorrhage and in mild iron deficiency anaemia (reactive thrombocytosis).

MCQs

1 Most patients with idiopathic thrombocytopenic purpura eventually develop leukaemia.
2 In idiopathic thrombocytopenic purpura, bone marrow megakaryocytes are usually absent.
3 The risk of intracerebral haemorrhages increases markedly when platelets fall to below the normal range.
4 Severe iron deficiency should be included in the differential diagnosis of thrombocytopenia.
5 Platelet formation is regulated by a hormone called erythropoietin.

Case 9
Anorexia, weight loss and vomiting

History

A 75-year-old housewife, who had no significant past medical history, was seen in accident and emergency with a 6-month history of increasing lethargy, anorexia, nausea and vomiting, itching and weight loss complicated by recurrent chest infections. On several occasions, she had been reassured by her doctor that 'her immune system had been affected by virus infections' and that it was this that had caused her to be so unwell for so long. Despite the reassurances and several courses of antibiotics, she continued to lose weight and was eventually sent to hospital with dehydration and reduced conscious level.

Initial investigations revealed a creatinine of $648\,\mu mol\,L^{-1}$ (normal range $<120\,\mu mol\,L^{-1}$) and a urea of $20.3\,mmol\,L^{-1}$ ($3–7\,mmol\,L^{-1}$). Her corrected calcium was $2.4\,mmol\,L^{-1}$ ($2.12–2.62\,mmol\,L^{-1}$) and her haemoglobin $8.8\,g\,dL^{-1}$ ($12–15\,g\,dL^{-1}$), with a white cell count of $6.8\times10^9\,L^{-1}$ ($(4–11)\times10^9\,L^{-1}$) and platelet count of $402\times10^9\,L^{-1}$ ($(150–400)\times10^9\,L^{-1}$). Plasma cells were seen on the blood film.

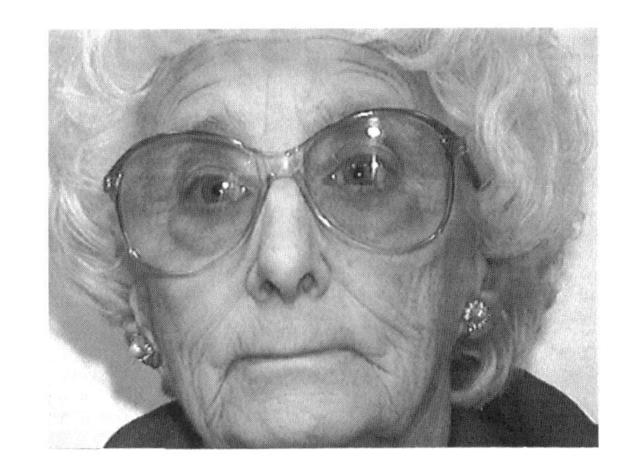

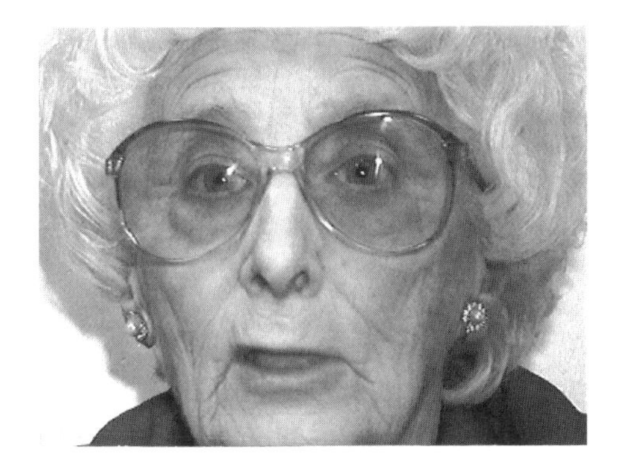

Notes

A skeletal survey showed multiple 'punched-out' radiolucencies. An immunoglobulin (Ig) screen was carried out and showed an IgA of $0.4\,g\,L^{-1}$ (0.8–4), IgG of $19.7\,g\,L^{-1}$ (5.3–16.5) and IgM of $0.4\,g\,L^{-1}$ (0.5–2). The diagnosis, IgG myeloma, was confirmed by bone marrow aspiration.

Myeloma is a malignant proliferation of the terminally differentiated, antibody-secreting form of B cells known as plasma cells. The disease occurs mostly in the elderly, with a mean age at diagnosis of 60 years. It is characterized by an increase in plasma cells in the bone marrow, lytic lesions in bones and the presence of a paraprotein (monoclonal antibody fragment) in the urine (as Bence-Jones protein) and/or serum. Renal failure is present at diagnosis in 15–20% of patients and 30% are hypercalcaemic. During the course of the disease, up to 50% of patients develop renal failure, often attributed to hypercalcaemia, dehydration, excretion of immunoglobulin light chains, renal infection or amyloid. In addition to hypercalcaemia, hyperviscosity syndrome, characterized by headaches, drowsiness, vertigo, deafness, visual disturbances, mucosal and intracranial bleeding, heart failure, fits and coma, can occur, particularly when the paraproteins are able to polymerize as they do in some IgA and IgG myelomas. At the present time, myeloma cannot be cured. Poor prognostic signs at diagnosis include a urea level of greater than $10\,mmol\,L^{-1}$, a haemoglobin level of less than $7.5\,g\,dL^{-1}$ and, most important, raised serum levels of β_2-microglobulin.

Basic science

Hypercalcaemia

Hypercalcaemia is thought to be essentially asymptomatic when modest ($<3\,mmol\,L^{-1}$) but, at higher levels, causes fatigue and depression, polyuria, polydipsia and dehydration, constipation, headaches and muscular aches and pains. Hypercalcaemia decreases the plateau phase of the cardiac action potential, which leads to a shortened heart rate-corrected Q–T interval (the time from the beginning of the QRS complex to the beginning of the T wave). Dysrhythmias are uncommon, but acute hypercalcaemia can be associated with bradycardia, first degree heart block (P–R interval $>0.2\,s$) and hypertension.

Primary hyperparathyroidism, the production of parathyroid hormone-related peptide (PTHRP) from solid tumours, and so-called 'calcaemic factors' from haematological malignancies such as myeloma account for most cases of hypercalcaemia seen. Malignancy-associated hypercalcaemia does not imply the presence of bone metastases (with the exception of breast cancer). Vitamin D intoxication, sarcoidosis, hyperthyroidism and Addison's disease are relatively rare causes of hypercalcaemia. Emergency treatment centres around vigorous rehydration with saline and administration of bisphosphonates and glucocorticoids pending treatment of the primary problem.

MCQs

1 Myeloma is a malignant proliferation of T lymphocytes.
2 Typical complications of myeloma are renal failure, anaemia and hypercalcaemia.
3 Severe hypercalcaemia causes constipation and oliguria.
4 Hypercalcaemia is associated with a shortened Q–T interval.
5 Most cases of malignancy-induced hypercalcaemia are associated with bone metastases.

Case 10
The man who developed calf pain on exercise

History

A 53-year-old labourer was admitted to hospital with a 6-month history of pain in his right calf on exercise. This typically came on after he had walked 100 m on the level, but would appear more quickly on ascending hills, and took a few minutes to go after he sat down to rest. For several months this had not proved to be too much of a problem, but he had, in the last few weeks, begun to notice that the same pain would wake him at night. He otherwise considered himself fit and well, although he had smoked since the age of 14 years and continued to smoke 30 cigarettes daily.

On examination, his foot pulses were palpable on the left, but absent on the right. A bruit was audible on auscultation of both femoral arteries.

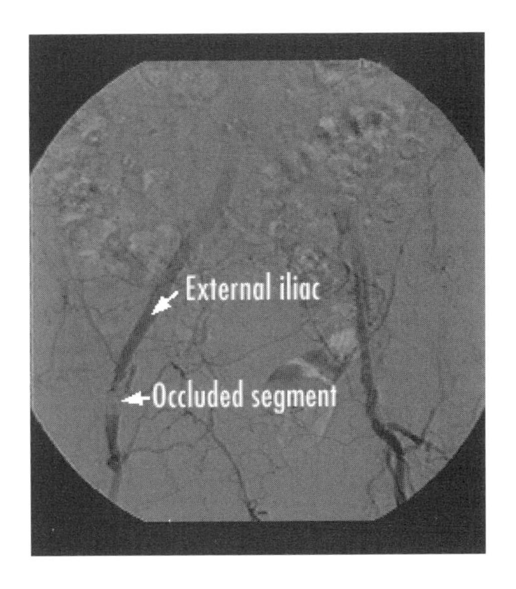

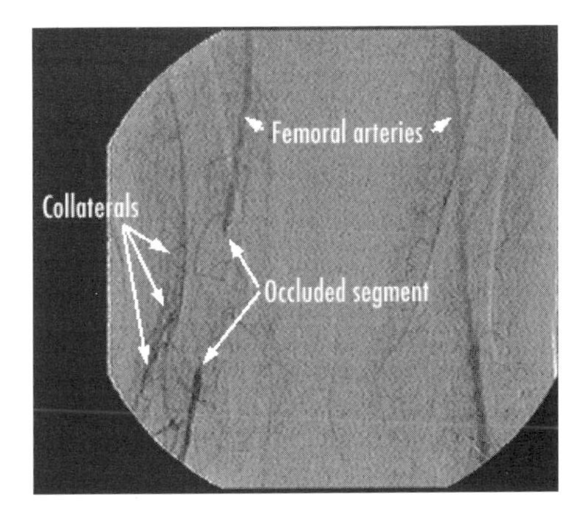

Notes

The patient had intermittent claudication due to atherosclerotic vascular occlusion.

Pain caused by insufficient oxygen reaching the muscles of the limbs is usually a result of atherosclerotic arterial disease. It is more common in men, increases with age and affects ≈2% of elderly people and 20% of those with arterial disease in the lower limbs. The prevalence of intermittent claudication in men aged 50–75 years is between 1% and 7%. The course of intermittent claudication (unlike critical ischaemia) is generally benign, with fewer than 25% of patients requiring surgical intervention. Nevertheless, as most people who have intermittent claudication have arterial insufficiency elsewhere, their mortality rate (15% over 5 years) is twice to three times that of age-matched controls, with ≥50% of deaths attributable to ischaemic heart disease.

Intermittent claudication is almost entirely confined to people who smoke or who are diabetic or hypertensive. The association of hypercholesterolaemia with peripheral vascular disease is not as clear.

Patients typically present with a chronic history of pain in the buttock or calf on exercise that is relieved by rest. More severe

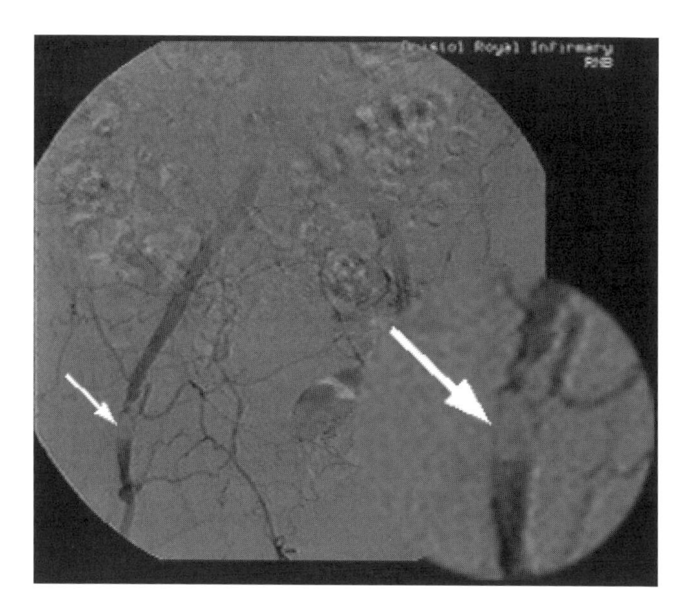

ischaemia leads to continuous pain in the foot, particularly when the limb is raised, such as when the patient is recumbent at night. Ultimately, ischaemic tissue loss and gangrene occur. Involvement of the aorta and/or the common iliac arteries may reduce internal pudendal blood flow and lead to impotence. Acute ischaemia, characterized by the acute onset of intermittent claudication, pain at rest or the development of a white, paralysed leg, is much less common than is progression to critical ischaemia in a chronically ischaemic limb.

Patients with intermittent claudication should be advised to take aspirin, stop smoking and walk for 30 min at least three times per week. Diabetes should be well controlled and hypertension treated (avoiding β-blockers). This is particularly important as, in diabetic patients, the presence of more distal disease is often less amenable to surgical intervention.

Basic science

Atherosclerotic plaque formation

The process of atherosclerotic plaque formation starts with damage to the endothelial cells that line arteries. Low density lipoproteins (LDLs) accumulate at the site and attract monocytes, which phagocytose the LDLs and become foam cells. The release of growth factors from adherent platelets stimulates smooth muscle cell migration from the media, and subsequent collagen formation results in the production of a fibrous plaque. Rupture of the plaque surface exposes a highly thrombogenic matrix, resulting in rapid occlusion of the already narrowed artery by platelets and thrombus. The mechanism of action of lowered circulating LDL cholesterol seems to be atherosclerotic plaque stabilization (resistance to rupture) rather than reduction in plaque size and increased vessel patency *per se*. Somewhat paradoxically, younger, softer plaques are more likely to fissure and result in acute coronary artery occlusion.

Blood vessel structure

Blood vessels may be categorized into:

1 Elastic arteries: these are thick-walled arteries that form the aorta and major blood vessels carrying blood away from the heart. Their large calibre and the laminar or spiral pattern of blood flow within them minimize turbulence and resistance. To withstand and smooth the peaks and troughs of pulsatile flow, their walls contain elastic connective tissue sheets interspersed with layers of smooth muscle cells that are able to recoil after each pulse. They do not actively vasoconstrict to a significant extent.

2 Smaller muscular arteries: these range down to about 0.3 mm in luminal diameter. They are relatively rich in smooth muscle and, as they contain less elastin than the main conducting arteries, their distensibility is reduced. These factors and their smaller luminal diameter give them considerably more active influence over blood flow.

3 Arterioles: these range from 0.3 mm to 10 μm in diameter, have a thin or even single layer of smooth muscle cells with occasional elastic fibres. Fluctuations in arteriole diameter govern minute to minute variation in capillary blood flow.

4 Capillaries (of which there are three kinds): these are the smallest blood vessels. Each measures around 1 mm in length, has a luminal diameter of 8–10 μm and often has its entire circumference formed by single endothelial cells. Most tissues have a rich capillary supply, but tendons and ligaments are poorly vascularized, cartilage and epithelia receive nutrients from blood vessels in neighbouring tissues and the cornea is entirely avascular, receiving nutrients only from the aqueous humour.

- 'Continuous capillaries' are fashioned from endothelial cells that form a lining interrupted only by small intercellular clefts between the tight junctions. The continuous capillaries that form the blood–brain barrier are distinct in that the endothelial cell perimeter is bounded entirely by tight junctions.
- Fenestrated capillaries are formed from fenestrated endothelial cells. Although most fenestrations are occluded by a delicate diaphragm, these capillaries are much more permeable to fluids and solutes than continuous capillaries. Fenestrated capillaries are found in the small intestine, where digested nutrients enter the bloodstream, and also in many endocrine glands to allow hormones rapid access to the bloodstream.
- Sinusoidal capillaries (also known as sinusoids) are highly specialized, very permeable capillaries with large irregular lumens, many fenestrations or even discontinuities of the wall and few tight junctions, and are found in the liver, lymphoid tissues, bone marrow and some endocrine organs. Large molecules and blood cells are able to pass from the capillary into surrounding tissues.

5 Postcapillary venules: 8–100 μm in diameter, formed when capillaries unite. They consist almost entirely of endothelium and are very permeable.

6 Veins: these have thicker connective tissue walls with little smooth muscle or elastin. Their large calibre ensures that, under normal conditions, 65% of circulating blood volume is in the venous 'capacitance' vessels at any one time. Venous pressure is low, their walls are correspondingly thinner than arteries of similar size and, in many, valves are present to aid the return of blood to the heart.

7 Cerebral venous sinuses and the venous sinuses of the heart: these are very thin-walled veins supported by surrounding tissues.

MCQs

1 More than 50% of patients with intermittent claudication die of ischaemic heart disease.
2 Once intermittent claudication is evident, stopping smoking has little effect on outcome.
3 All tissues in the body receive a capillary blood supply.
4 Fenestrated capillaries are typically found in the blood–brain barrier.
5 Postcapillary venules, unlike capillaries, are almost impermeable to fluid and salts.

Case 11
A boring television show

History

A 73-year-old woman with no previous medical history sat down to watch the television and drifted off to sleep. The next thing she knew, her husband was trying to rouse her by tapping gently on her cheek. She felt well in herself and, although somewhat tired, thought that the sole cause of her somnolence was a particularly boring programme on television. Nevertheless, her family insisted that she see her doctor and an urgent appointment was made. On examination in clinic, the patient's blood pressure was 146/74 mmHg, her heart sounds were normal and she was found to be well perfused with no evidence of congestive cardiac failure. Her ankle reflexes were brisk and her sublingual temperature was 36.2 °C. The chief finding of note was a bradycardia at 35 beats per minute (b.p.m.). She was referred to accident and emergency with a presumptive diagnosis that was confirmed on her **ECG**.

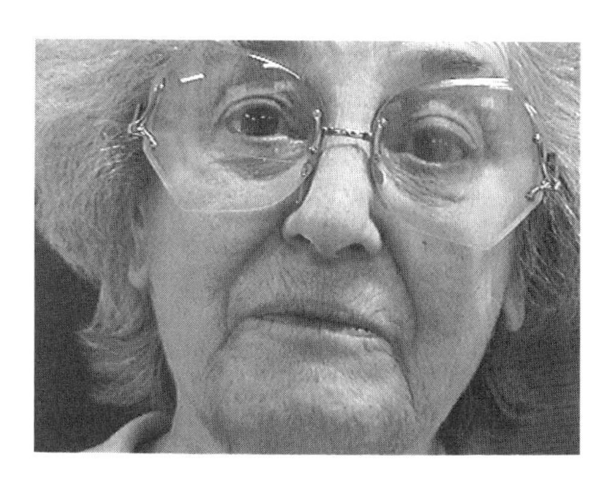

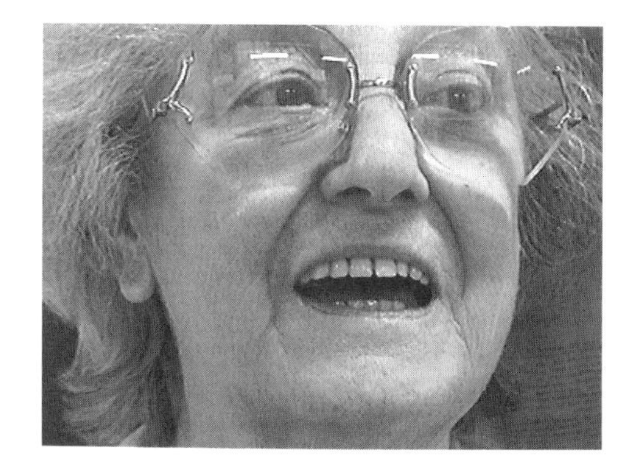

Notes

The ECG showed bradycardia secondary to complete heart block.

The patient was taken immediately to the catheter laboratory and a permanent pacemaker was installed. A further **ECG** was recorded immediately after insertion of the device.

In complete heart block, no atrial impulses are conducted to the ventricles. As all of the supraventricular impulses are blocked within the conducting system, the ventricles are activated by a subsidiary ectopic escape pacemaker, either within the atrioventricular (AV) node or within the ventricles. If ventricular depolarization (and hence the QRS complex) is of normal duration and occurs at between 40 and 55 b.p.m. (escape rhythm), it is likely

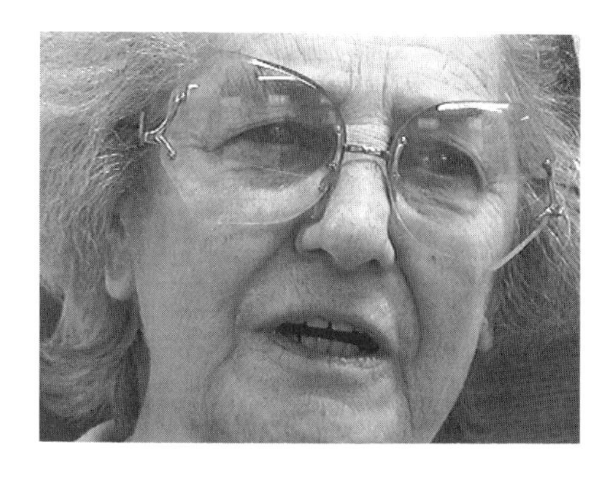

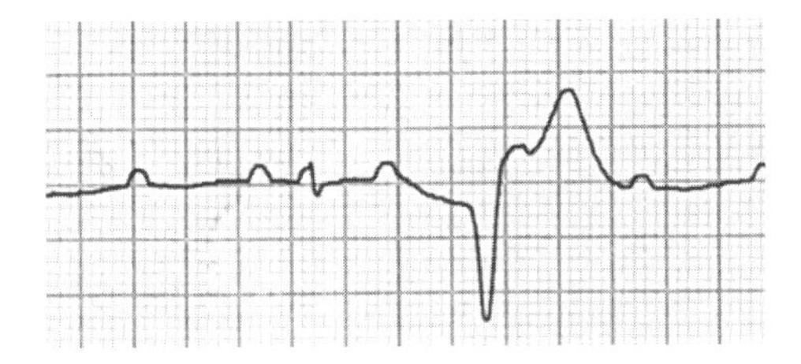

that the block is at the level of the AV node. If the origin of complete heart block is within or adjacent to the His bundle, the QRS complex is usually widened and the escape rate is ≤40 b.p.m. If the ventricular pacemaker is away from the His bundle, its intrinsic depolarization rate is around 30–35 b.p.m. and, as it is not influenced by parasympathetic tone, the rate is independent of exercise, breathing, emotions and anticholinergic drugs, such as atropine. As atrial depolarization is completely dissociated from ventricular depolarization, the P wave bears no relationship to the QRS complex. The idioventricular pacemaker may move from one part of the ventricle to another. A pause between the two may lead to a Stokes–Adams attack—syncope associated with temporary asystole.

Basic science

Causes of bradycardia

Bradycardia (a pulse rate of <50 b.p.m. in the doctor's surgery) is caused either by faulty conduction of cardiac impulses throughout the heart (complete heart block) or through slowed sinoatrial node impulse generation. If the latter occurs, and the rate slows to a level at which cells further down in the conducting system or within the ventricular walls are able to depolarize, escape rhythm appears, but may disappear again once the rate of sinoatrial node depolarization increases. Acute sinoatrial node malfunction can occur in the early stages of myocardial infarction, or may be related to hypothyroidism or drugs such as β-adrenoreceptor blockers or digoxin. In carotid sinus syndrome, stimulation of the carotid sinus in elderly patients leads to inappropriately protracted and profound afferent discharges to the brain stem (nucleus tractus solitarius). The resulting loss of sympathetic tone causes marked bradycardia or sinus arrest and drop attacks, in which the patient may lose consciousness so briefly that he/she denies it and attributes a facial injury or fractured hip to a fall.

Causes of bradycardia

Sinus bradycardia
Sinus arrest—Stokes–Adams attacks
Sick sinus syndrome
Sinoatrial block
Myocardial infarction
Carotid sinus syndrome
Complete heart block
Drugs (digoxin, morphine, β-blockers)
Hypothyroidism
Hypothermia
Raised intracranial pressure
Rapid rise in blood pressure
Vasovagal attack (transient increase in vagal tone, e.g. vomiting)
Physical training (normal)
Jaundice

Causes of tachycardia

Sinus tachycardia
- Exercise
- Anxiety
- Hyperthyroidism
- Congestive cardiac failure
- Drugs (atropine, adrenaline, vasodilators, β_1-stimulants)
- Hypovolaemia (shock)

Supraventricular tachycardia
Atrial fibrillation
Atrial flutter with 2 : 1 block
Ventricular tachycardia

MCQs

1 In complete heart block, only some atrial impulses reach the ventricles.
2 In complete heart block, the ventricular rate may be increased by exercise.
3 In carotid sinus syndrome, fleeting loss of consciousness may occur.
4 Vomiting is typically associated with tachycardia.
5 Spontaneous changes in pacemaker location in complete heart block may lead to syncope.

Case 12
A chance finding at a medical

History

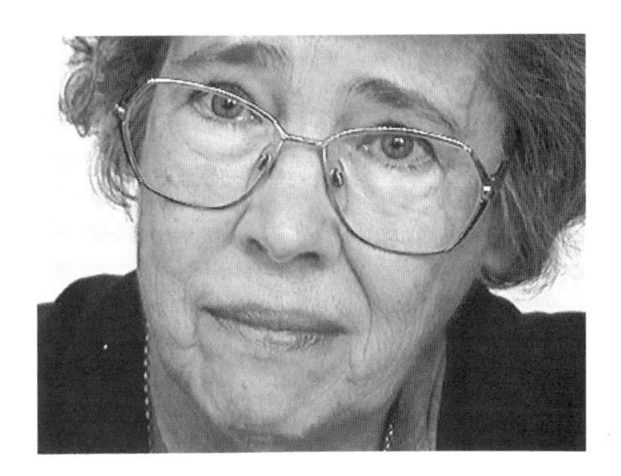

A 55-year-old housewife, with a history of hypertension since the birth of her first child 33 years previously, was seen by her GP for a repeat prescription for β-blockers. For some time, she had noticed that, when out walking with friends, particularly in the evening, she would find herself a little breathless and 'tight in the throat'. She attributed these symptoms to her antihypertensive medication and did not report them until a routine cholesterol check (13 mmol L^{-1}, 505 mg/100 mL!) prompted her doctor to ask some more direct questions. There were no signs of hyperlipidaemia on examination.

Notes

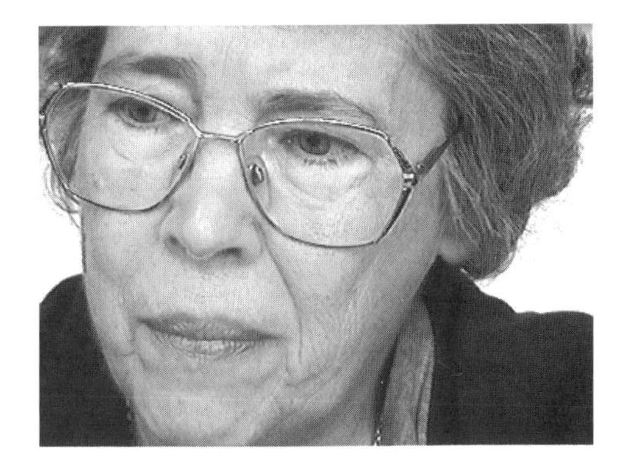

The patient had hypercholesterolaemia and ischaemic heart disease. Direct questioning elicited a history typical of angina with chest pain on exertion and relieved by rest. She was prescribed an HMGCoA-reductase inhibitor, despite which, several years later, she developed unstable angina and then a full myocardial infarction. The patient had a past history of rheumatoid arthritis, but did not smoke and did not have diabetes or a family history of ischaemic heart disease.

Basic science

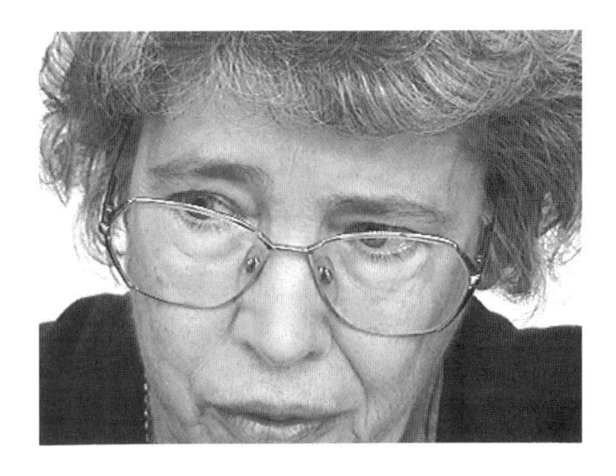

Lipids are used principally as a medium of energy storage and as thermal insulation. They are also required for the synthesis of steroid hormones, bile salts and cell membranes. The relatively high fat western diet and inherited metabolic defects that predispose to high levels of circulating cholesterol are heavily implicated in coronary heart disease, which accounts for 30% of deaths in men and 25%

of deaths in women, and, to a lesser extent, with cerebrovascular disease and peripheral vascular disease. The absolute risk of increased circulating cholesterol is such that increased levels of low density lipoprotein (LDL) cholesterol and decreased levels of high density lipoprotein (HDL) cholesterol are more strongly associated with cardiovascular risk in diabetics than is either smoking or hypertension. There is clear epidemiological evidence of the benefits of treating hyperlipidaemia in the prevention of coronary heart disease.

Pain derived from myocardial ischaemia

The heavy, squeezing or crushing central chest pain described by people with myocardial infarction is similar to that of angina pectoris, but is more severe, lasts longer and is more often associated with agitation, sweating and nausea. In about one-third of cases, the pain radiates to the arms. Pain radiating to the neck and lower jaw, although less common, is very characteristic of the pain of myocardial ischaemia and more specific. Asymptomatic coronary artery disease and silent ischaemia on treadmill testing are present in 2–4% of middle-aged men. In patients with known

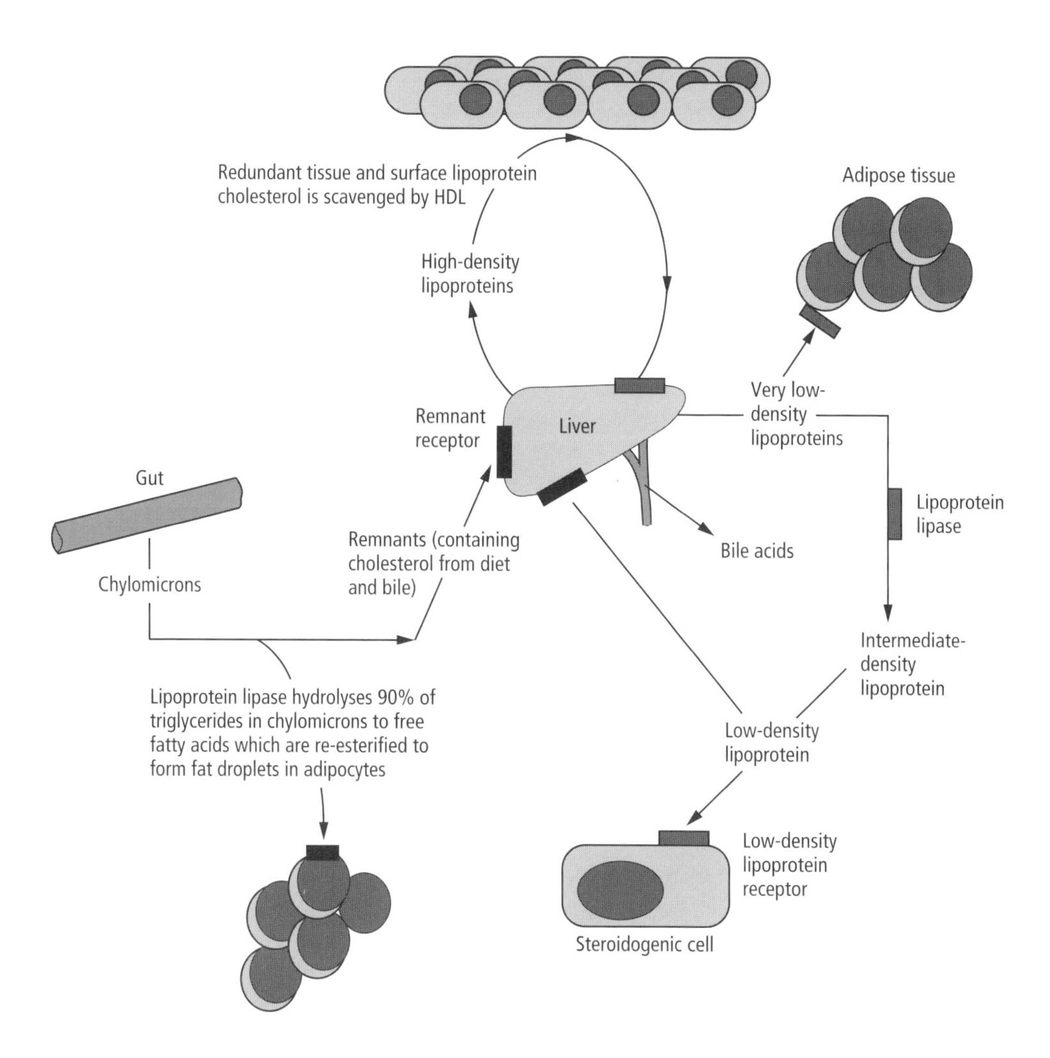

coronary artery disease, one-third are said to have recorded positive treadmill tests without any associated pain. In patients with angina pectoris, ischaemic events are completely painless at least 40% of the time. Taking all patients together, 20–30% of myocardial infarctions are painless, and this figure is higher in diabetics and in patients over the age of 65 years.

MCQs

1 In diabetics, smoking is more strongly associated with cardiovascular disease than is hypercholesterolaemia.
2 LDL receptors hydrolyse triglycerides to free fatty acids.
3 Free fatty acids are re-esterified in adipocytes to fat droplets.
4 In the developed world, coronary heart disease causes 40% of all deaths.
5 HDL cholesterol levels are inversely correlated with coronary heart disease risk.

Case 13
Breathlessness at night

History

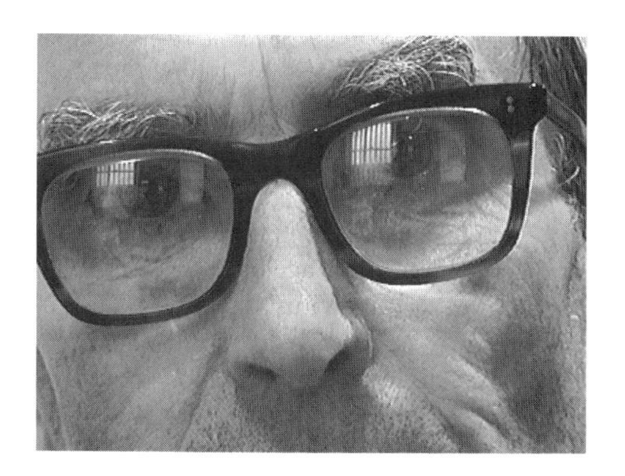

A 62-year-old man was seen in clinic with a 2-month history of being woken with increasing frequency by shortness of breath. When this happened, he would be forced to sit upright on the bed for 10 min or more to get his breath back, and found that it helped to open the window to let cool air in. He also complained of mild ankle swelling and shortness of breath on exertion.

At the age of 8 years, he had developed involuntary jerking movements of the right upper limb and had been kept off school for over 18 months. Subsequently, he was always considered 'delicate' and was not allowed to do physical exercise. Unfortunately, his lack of education led to a working life as a labourer, which he believes exacerbated his condition. Some 20 years after his original illness, a prosthetic heart valve was inserted and, 10 years after that, recurrent episodes of breathlessness and palpitations were relieved by the insertion of a pacemaker.

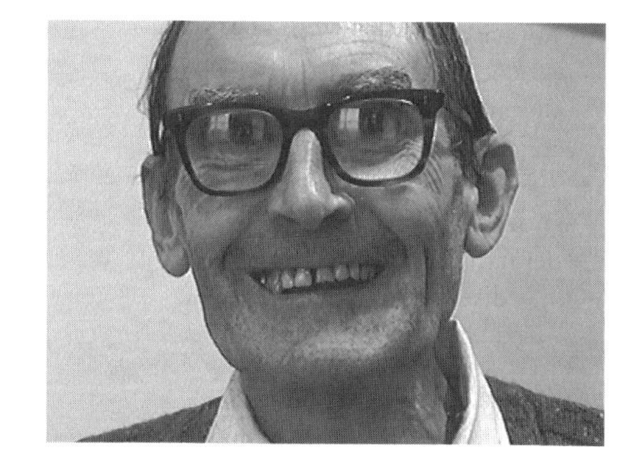

He had smoked 5–10 cigarettes daily since his teenage years, and suffered from recurrent attacks of bronchitis, but drank very little alcohol.

On examination, his blood pressure was 144/96 mmHg and his pulse was regular, with occasional ectopic beats, at a rate of 100 beats per minute (b.p.m.). His **jugular venous pressure** (JVP) was raised 5 cm, and there was mild peripheral and sacral **oedema**. His apex beat was displaced to the anterior axillary line (fifth interspace), and a pacemaker was palpable in the upper left chest wall. A prosthetic click at the beginning of systole was audible from the end of the bed. Auscultation revealed heart sounds consistent with the presence of a mitral ball valve and mid- to late-inspiratory crackles at both bases.

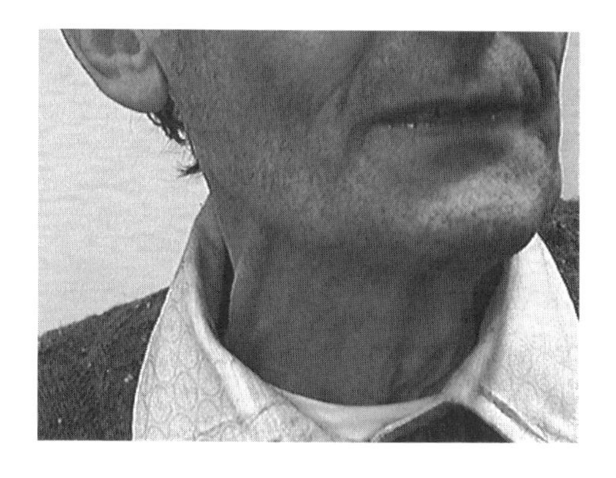

A chest X-ray confirmed the presence of the pacemaker and mitral valve replacement. The heart was considerably enlarged (18 cm in the maximum transverse dimension) and septal lines indicated mild pulmonary oedema. An echocardiogram showed a dilated heart with a globally poorly contracting left ventricle.

Notes

The patient had a number of late manifestations of rheumatic heart disease, having had rheumatic fever at the age of 8 years. His presentation with Saint Vitus' dance, also known as Sydenham's chorea, was misdiagnosed by his teachers at the time as a case of 'playing the fool'.

Rheumatic fever is an acute febrile systemic disorder affecting particularly the heart and joints, but also the skin, subcutaneous tissue and central nervous system, that follows infection with Lancefield group A β-haemolytic streptococci. Acute rheumatic carditis was a major cause of acute myocardial damage and heart failure in young patients worldwide in the earlier part of this century, and remains a major cause of morbidity and mortality in poorer nations.

The disease causes a pancarditis characterized by pericarditis, myocarditis and endocarditis.

Rheumatic pericarditis is characterized by a serofibrinous pericardial effusion and friction rub.

Rheumatic myocarditis is characterized acutely by tachycardia, cardiomegaly and/or heart failure, with granuloma formation (the pathognomonic Aschoff bodies) and scarring of the heart muscle itself.

Rheumatic endocarditis is characterized acutely by the development of a transient mitral diastolic murmur (described by Carey–Coombs) caused by blood flowing across inflamed leaflets. Endocarditis subsequently leads to fibrous thickening and adhesions that chronically and progressively impair valvular function.

The diagnosis is made on the basis of the presence of at least one so-called major and two minor criteria, or two major criteria if previous streptococcal infection can be shown to have occurred. The major criteria are:
- Sydenham's chorea,
- erythema marginatum,
- subcutaneous nodules,
- flitting polyarthropathy, and
- carditis,

while the minor criteria are:
- fever,
- tender joints,
- raised inflammatory indices,
- a positive throat swab,
- raised white count, and
- first degree heart block.

Basic science

Heart failure

In general, heart failure is caused by direct myocardial damage (typically ischaemic),

Table 13.1 Causes of heart failure

Damage to the myocardium	Volume overload
• Coronary artery disease (myocardial ischaemia) • Toxins (alcohol) • Cardiomyopathies • Myocarditis	• Mitral regurgitation • Aortic regurgitation • Atrial septal defect • Ventricular septal defect (postinfarction)
Pressure overload	**Impaired ventricular filling**
• Hypertension • Aortic stenosis • Coarctation of the aorta	• Mitral stenosis • Constrictive pericarditis • Hypertrophic cardiomyopathy • Restrictive cardiomyopathy • Atrial myxoma • Tachyarrhythmias

volume or pressure overload (typically valvular regurgitation or stenosis) or impaired ventricular filling.

Precipitating causes include dysrhythmias (such as uncontrolled tachycardias and, particularly, atrial fibrillation with a rapid ventricular response), thyrotoxicosis (which has a direct myocardial as well as a volume overload effect), anaemia and infections. The inappropriate use of calcium antagonists, β-blockers or one of the many antiarrhythmic drugs that are negatively inotropic, such as disopyramide, may also sometimes be responsible for heart failure. Sudden onset of acute heart failure is typically caused by a myocardial infarction or the onset of a dysrhythmia such as atrial fibrillation.

Typical symptoms of heart failure are breathlessness, tiredness, fatigue and swollen ankles. Patients often complain of a wheeze or cough at night, and frequently need to sit out of bed and open windows to ease orthopnoea and paroxysmal nocturnal dyspnoea. Physical signs of heart failure include sinus tachycardia, breathlessness, basal crackles and a third and/or fourth heart sound, ankle oedema, raised JVP, tender enlargement of the liver, heart murmurs, cardiomegaly and, occasionally, ascites.

Assuming that the underlying cause of heart failure has been addressed, treatments for chronic heart failure include general measures, such as stopping smoking and reducing salt intake, taking 1–2 units of alcohol daily (unless it was the primary cause of the problem), rest and therapy with diuretics, nitrates, angiotensin-converting enzyme inhibitors, calcium antagonists, digoxin and anticoagulants.

MCQs

1 Heart failure in rheumatic carditis can occur in the absence of valvular disease.
2 Pericardial involvement can lead to tamponade.
3 Excessive alcohol ingestion is a potentially reversible cause of heart failure.
4 Heart failure is often associated with Paget's disease of bone.
5 Sinus bradycardia is typically found on examination of patients with heart failure.

Case 14
Central chest pain

History

A 62-year-old domestic worker with non-insulin-dependent diabetes and a history of cigarette smoking was admitted to hospital with a 6-h history of severe (excruciating) central chest pain radiating to both axillae, associated with nausea and sweating. She had a previous history of angina that had, until the day of admission, responded rapidly and consistently to treatment with sublingual nitrates. On this occasion, the pain had persisted despite nitrates, and an ambulance had been called.

The findings of note on examination were a blood pressure of 162/94 mmHg with a regular pulse of 80 beats per minute. She was moderately tachypnoeic and, on auscultation of the chest, a few crackles and wheezes were noted. The changes were ascribed to chronic obstructive pulmonary disease. There were no signs of heart failure, and fundoscopy did not reveal any evidence of diabetic or hypertensive retinopathy. Total cholesterol, measured within 2 h of admission to hospital, was 6.2 mmol L^{-1} or 240 mg/100 mL and her HbA1c* was 9%. An **ECG** did not show any evidence of a myocardial infarction at the time of admission, and she was treated for unstable angina. Several days after admission, the severe pain recurred.

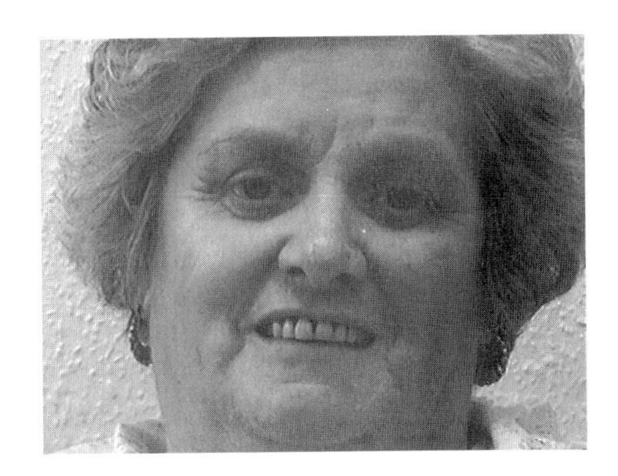

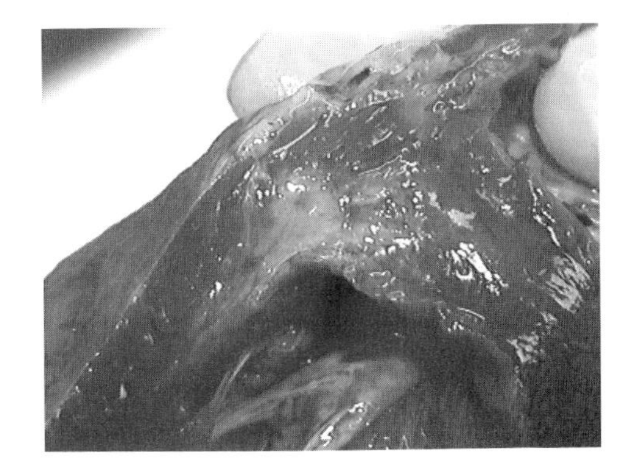

Notes

Despite ongoing intravenous treatment, after a short history of unstable angina, the patient suffered a myocardial infarction in hospital.

The prognosis of a myocardial infarction is largely determined by the events that take place within the first few hours. Potentially lethal rhythm disturbances can be treated and infarct size limited by restoring perfusion. Thrombolysis within 1 h of the onset of pain reduces mortality at 35 days by almost 40%. Thrombolytic therapy also limits **infarct** size and improves left ventricular function. After more than 12 h, only 0.5% of extra lives are saved by thrombolysis. Primary cor-

*HbA1c is a glycosylated haemoglobin. The percentage of glycosylated haemoglobin provides a fairly reliable representation of the mean blood glucose over the previous 6–12 weeks. The 'A1c' component of haemoglobin is chosen for technical reasons.

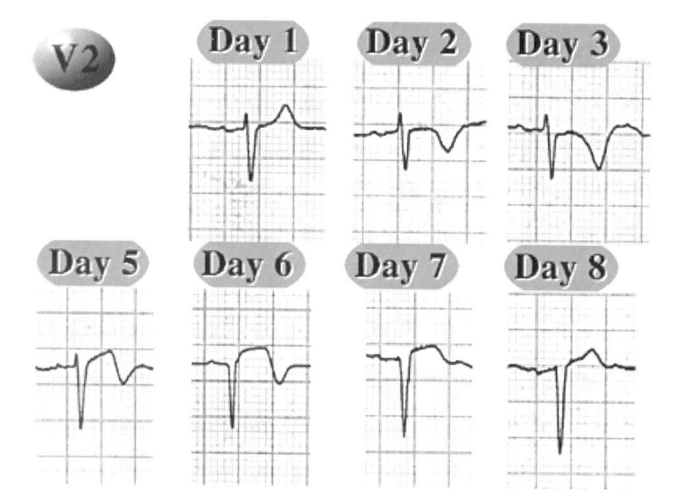

onary angioplasty in the average community hospital does not reduce deaths more than thrombolytic therapy, but costs considerably more. In this patient, although thrombolytic therapy did not prevent myocardial infarction, it may have prevented more extensive or lethal infarction.

Basic science

Complications of myocardial infarction

In general, the complications of myocardial infarction can be divided into electrical and mechanical. The most common cause of death within the first few minutes of the event is ventricular fibrillation, and no fewer than 90% of patients with acute myocardial infarction have some cardiac rhythm or conduction abnormality, some of which may be related to successful coronary artery reperfusion. Prompt coronary artery reperfusion is almost certainly responsible for the continuing fall in the incidence of other complications, such as rupture of the left ventricle, rupture of the intraventricular septum or papillary muscles and left ventricular aneurysm formation (observed in 10% of patients). Mural thrombus and pulmonary and systemic emboli, pericarditis and Dressler's syndrome (characterized by pleuropericardial chest pain and fever beginning a few days to 6 weeks after myocardial infarction) also occur, and other sequelae, such as cardiogenic shock in the short term, chronic left ventricular failure in the longer term and the many psychological sequelae of 'heart attacks', remain major problems.

Cardiovascular risk determinants

The British Regional Heart Study identified a simple calculation that can be used to identify those in the top quantile of risk.

If the following calculation exceeds 1000, the patient's risk is in the top 20%:

1 7.5 × number of years spent smoking,
2 plus 4.5 × systolic blood pressure (average of two readings),
3 plus 265 if a patient recalls a 'doctor's diagnosis of coronary heart disease',
4 plus 150 if the patient currently suffers chest pain on exertion,
5 plus 80 if a parent died of 'heart trouble',
6 plus 150 if the patient is diabetic.

The principal modifiable risk factors for coronary heart disease are:

- raised total cholesterol,
- hypertension,
- smoking,
- diabetes mellitus,
- obesity,

- lack of exercise,
- low high density lipoprotein (HDL) cholesterol, and
- high triglycerides.

Myocardial ischaemia

Please see 'Basic science' discussions of Cases 12 and 15.

MCQs

1 Dressler's syndrome typically develops 8–12 weeks after myocardial infarction.
2 In acute myocardial infarction, the earlier thrombolytic treatment is started, the greater the benefit.
3 Mural thrombosis can lead to further myocardial infarction.
4 Thrombolysis in acute myocardial infarction may itself be responsible for dysrhythmias.
5 Early thrombolysis reduces the incidence of ventricular aneurysm after acute myocardial infarction.

Case 15
Chest pain at rest

History

A 64-year-old project manager with a long history of exercise-induced chest pain was seen in accident and emergency with chest pain that failed to go away with rest. He had a family history of ischaemic heart disease and a personal history of the same. For several years after it first started, he had been able to predict the amount of exercise that he would be able to do—the distance that he would be able to walk uphill—before the onset of a feeling of a weight on his chest. Initially, the pain would only come on with exercise and he would be able to 'walk through it'. Subsequently, he found that he had to take 'a couple of squirts of GTN' (glyceryl trinitrate) and rest for a short while before the unpleasant sensation would pass off. In the month before he presented to casualty, he noticed that the exercise-induced pain came on more often and, on the day of admission, the pain appeared at rest and became gradually worse, even though he retired to bed to rest. Until 14 years previously, he had smoked 20 cigarettes and drank up to 3 pints of beer a day.

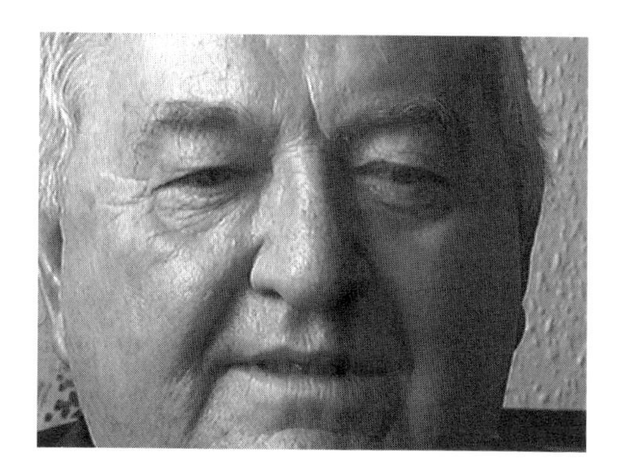

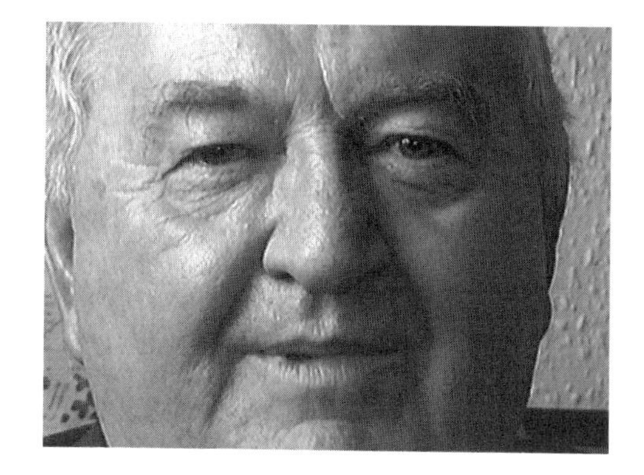

Notes

The patient had developed unstable angina on top of established ischaemic heart disease.

Unstable angina is defined as troublesome or frequent episodes of chest pain due to myocardial ischaemia that have appeared within the previous 4 weeks; angina that occurs recurrently at rest and lasts longer than 15 min (the sign with the greatest associated risk) or previously stable angina that increases in duration, frequency or severity. Unstable angina is an ominous diagnosis that requires prompt treatment to prevent progression to myocardial infarction and sudden death. Within the first 3 months of the diagnosis, sudden death occurs in 2% of patients and 10% have a myocardial infarction. Over the first year, these numbers rise to 10% and 15%, respectively. The mechanism that causes angina to become unstable appears to be qualitatively similar to that of myocardial infarction (i.e. decreased myocardial oxygen supply through decreased coronary artery blood flow), rather than increased myocardial oxygen demand that characterizes episodes of stable angina. The difference between unstable angina and myocardial infarction is therefore only the completeness of luminal obstruction or the duration of obstruction. This patient exhibited many typical features of angina pectoris: relatively stable, exercise-induced chest pain of a pressing or crushing nature, often radiating to the arm or neck, that resolves when the precipitating activity is stopped, and is hastened in its departure by rapidly absorbed nitrates, such as GTN. A heavy meal, walking uphill, cold weather, anxiety, walking against the wind and carrying heavy bags are typical precipitating factors.

Basic science

Causes of myocardial ischaemia

The most common cause of myocardial ischaemia is atherosclerosis in the coronary arteries. Coronary flow can also be limited by arterial emboli, coronary artery smooth muscle contraction (spasm) and arteritis. Increased oxygen demands of the myocardium (massive hypertrophy), decreased oxygen-carrying capacity of the blood (marked anaemia) and congenital anomalies in coronary artery structure can all exacerbate the effects of atherosclerotic narrowing of the coronary arteries, but are rarely the sole causes of myocardial ischaemia.

Coronary atherosclerosis is often present before the age of 20 years, and is widespread in later life. Narrowing of coronary vessels sufficient to cause silent myocardial ischaemia on exercise is also relatively common, and sudden coronary death is a frequent presenting manifestation of coronary disease.

MCQs

1 Within 3 months of the onset of unstable angina, 2% of patients have a myocardial infarction.
2 Unstable angina is precipitated by increased myocardial oxygen demand.
3 Walking uphill, cold weather, anxiety and fasting are typical angina precipitants.
4 Coronary artery spasm is a common cause of myocardial ischaemia.
5 Coronary atherosclerosis is not usually present on autopsy examination until after the age of 30 years.

Case 16
Fevers and chills

History

A 59-year-old housewife was admitted to hospital with a 5-day history of fevers and chills, diarrhoea, anorexia, dysphoria and profound lethargy. At the age of 7 years, she had suffered a severe attack of rheumatic fever followed by a succession of prolonged admissions to hospital. At the age of 23 years, the patient required a mitral valvotomy and, at the age of 30 years, the mitral valve was replaced with a Starr–Edwards ball valve which, unfortunately, produced only modest symptomatic benefits. For the two decades that followed the patient remained reasonably well, although her exercise tolerance was very limited and she continued to be bothered by the loud noise of the valve. Five days before her current admission to hospital, she began to become even more tired, complained of feeling alternatively cold and shaky then hot and sweaty, and described 'electric shock sensations', abdominal pain and feelings of impending doom.

On examination, her temperature was 38.2 °C and her pulse rate was 104 beats per minute with a blood pressure of 110/66 mmHg. A mixed aortic valve murmur was audible in addition to prosthetic sounds on auscultation of the chest. The apex beat was displaced into the mid-axillary line, and there was evidence of congestive cardiac failure. A number of splinter haemorrhages were seen.

Notes

The patient had developed infective endocarditis.

Infective endocarditis is an infection of the heart valves or endocardium. It usually occurs on abnormal structures, and may follow an acute or chronic course depending on the organism involved. Classical symptoms are:

- fever,
- cardiac murmurs,
- weight loss,
- malaise and anorexia, and
- embolic manifestations such as splinter haemorrhages.

More chronic features, such as finger clubbing, Osler's nodes in the finger pulp, Roth's spot on the retina, splenomegaly, anaemia and haematuria, are less commonly seen.

In all cases, the causative organism is spilled into the blood on a continuous basis, and

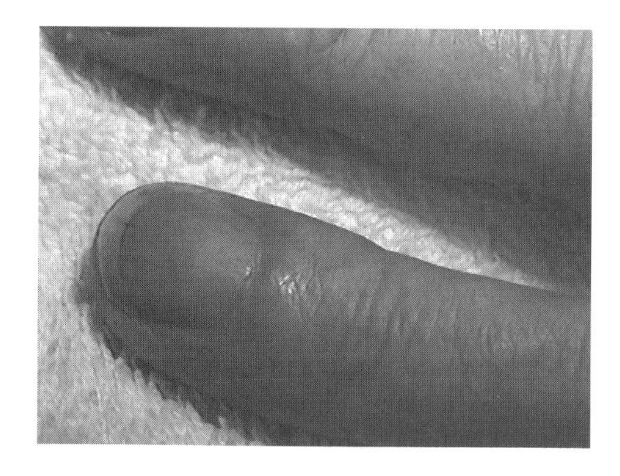

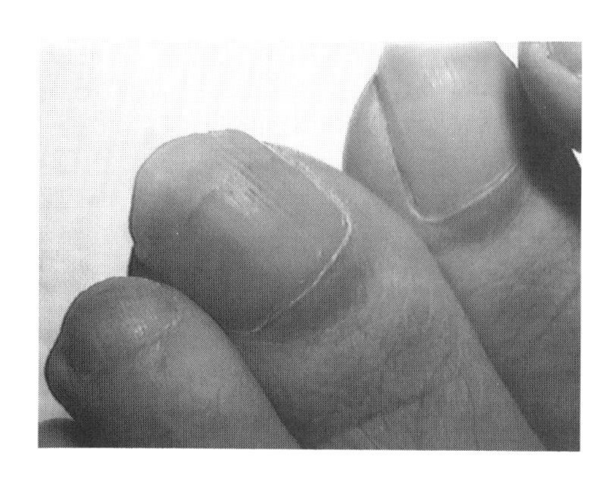

should be detectable on culture unless antimicrobial therapy has recently been used or is currently in use. Embolization of friable fibrin vegetations can cause pulmonary, brain, renal, heart, gastrointestinal or peripheral infarction depending on the site of the infection, and destruction of the valves can necessitate urgent surgical intervention.

Basic science

Pyrexia of unknown origin

The presence of bacterial endocarditis may be difficult to recognize in middle-aged and elderly patients in whom the significance of a heart murmur and a modest fever may be overlooked. Heart murmurs are often absent altogether in intravenous drug users who develop bacterial endocarditis with vegetations on the tricuspid valve and, in all groups, prior exposure to antibiotics may render initial blood cultures negative and further obscure the diagnosis.

The term pyrexia or fever of unknown origin (PUO) is usually applied when clinical examination and the usual diagnostic tests, such as bacteriological investigation of blood or other body fluids, biochemical and haematological investigation and scans, have failed to identify the cause. Infections which were once responsible for the majority of cases of PUO are now implicated in fewer than 40% of cases and, in many of these, it is the presentation rather than the causative organism that turns out to be unusual.

In the western world, the more common causes of PUO include tumours, such as carcinoma and Hodgkin's disease, connective tissue disorders, hypersensitivity reactions and infections, principally tuberculosis. Tuberculosis in these cases is usually extrapulmonary and, in overwhelming infection, skin tests may be negative.

Septic shock

Septic shock is bacteraemia-induced failure of tissue perfusion. Characteristic clinical features are hypotension, oliguria, tachycardia, tachypnoea and fever, and the usual cause is endotoxin release from Gram-negative enteric organisms. Often, the causative organism is a commensal that has spread from a contiguous site, such as the gastrointestinal tract, biliary tree or perineum, but, in immunosuppressed patients or following a burn, the lungs or skin are often implicated as entry sites. Predisposing factors are myeloproliferative and neoplastic disorders, immunosuppression, hepatic cirrhosis and diabetes mellitus, often in hospitalized patients who have undergone an invasive procedure. Most at risk are young women and people at the extremes of age.

Toxins from bacterial cell walls activate the complement and coagulation systems to alter the microvascular blood flow, injure cells and induce intravascular coagulation. The release of vasoactive peptides causes microvascular leakage, peripheral pooling in capillary beds and circulatory collapse. The kidneys and lungs are particularly susceptible to the early effects of endotoxin release. Failure of perfusion of the skin and viscera, together with the shunting of blood and possible failure of utilization of available oxygen, leads to profound acidosis and irreversible sequelae.

MCQs

1 Myocardial infarction is a complication of bacterial endocarditis.
2 In bacterial endocarditis, surgery is contraindicated until the infection is cured.
3 An oral temperature of less than 36 °C can be normal.
4 Body temperature is increased in the second half (luteal phase) of the menstrual cycle.
5 Hyperthermia associated with infections is due in part to the release of interleukin-1.

Case 17
The man who was so tired he could cry

History

A 78-year-old former bank manager presented to his doctor with non-specific tiredness and mild breathlessness. His health had previously been exemplary apart from occasional chest infections and, until the trouble began, he had continued to maintain his house, captain the local bowls team and tend his immaculate garden as well as he had done since his retirement. Seven weeks previously he noticed that he felt more tired than usual. He suspected that 'he was just getting old', but decided to seek his doctor's advice in case he was developing a chest infection similar to the one that he had suffered 3 months previously. At that time, he was found to have a blood pressure of 168/100 mmHg with a regular pulse of 80 beats per minute (b.p.m.). On this occasion, his pulse was 130 b.p.m. and irregular, with a blood pressure of 146/98 mmHg and normal heart sounds. He was referred to hospital.

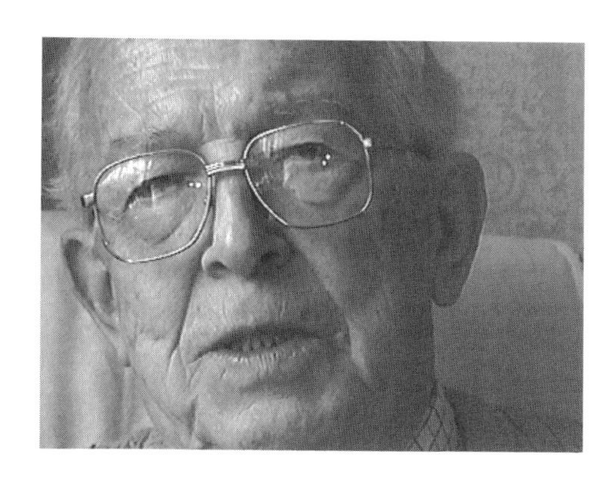

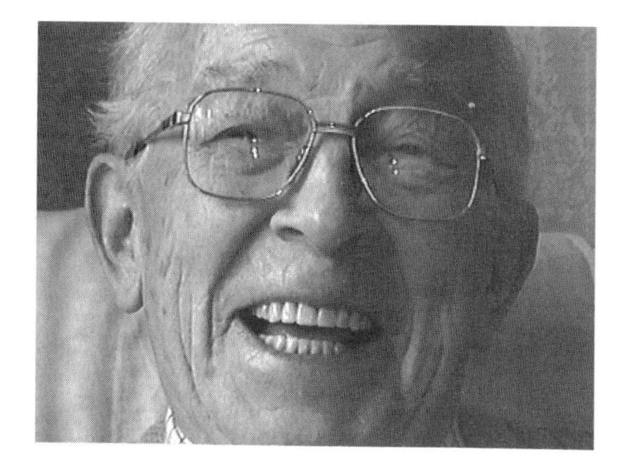

Notes

The patient had developed atrial fibrillation. An **ECG** showed a fast ventricular response to atrial fibrillation, but no evidence of ischaemia. He was cardioverted electrically, but, at review 6 weeks later, was found to have reverted to atrial fibrillation once again.

Chest X-ray showed mild pulmonary oedema and cardiomegaly. An echocardiogram showed normal mitral valve cusps, mild mitral regurgitation and moderately impaired left ventricular function. The left atrium was dilated to 7 cm in diameter. His liver function tests, including γ-glutamyl transpeptidase (γ-GT) level, were within normal limits, and his thyroid-stimulating hormone (TSH) level was $1.5\,\mathrm{mU\,L^{-1}}$ (normal range = 0.5–$5\,\mathrm{mU\,L^{-1}}$).

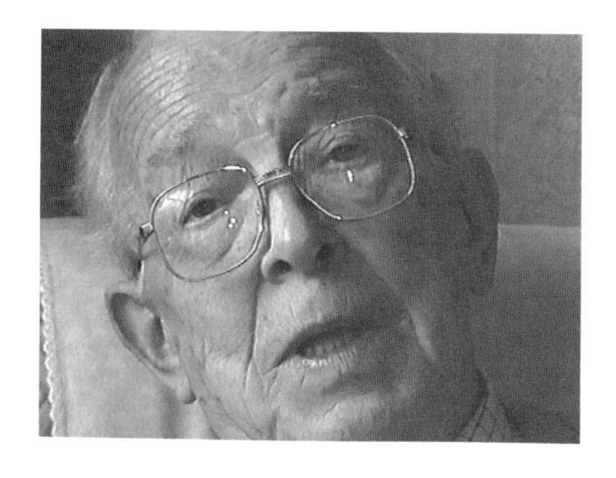

Atrial fibrillation is the commonest sustained cardiac dysrhythmia, increasing in prevalence from 0.5% of patients under 60 years of age to 11.6% of those over 75 years. The loss of synchronized atrial contraction reduces cardiac output by 10–50%, reduces exercise tolerance, predisposes to systemic embolization and can cause breathlessness. It is a non-specific response to atrial distension seen after pulmonary embolism and in 10–15% of myocardial infarctions. Thyrotoxicosis and alcoholic cardiomyopathy are associated with atrial fibrillation, and the condition is often chronic and progressive in hypertensive heart disease, mitral valve disease and heart failure. The duration of atrial fibrillation and the size of the left atrium on echocardiography predict the success of electrical cardioversion, with short duration and normal architecture predicting the greatest chance of success.

The rate of spontaneous cardioversion when atrial fibrillation is of short duration (≤6 h) is 35%, and almost 50% at 8 h. In acute atrial fibrillation of less than 3 days' duration, 2 mg kg^{-1} flecainide (maximum 150 mg) intravenously (i.v.) over 10 min (with ECG monitoring) restores sinus rhythm in more than 90% of patients. Cardioversion in atrial fibrillation of more than 48 h duration carries a risk of thromboembolism of 3–5%. The patient should therefore be anticoagulated for at least 3–4 weeks before cardioversion is attempted and for at least a month thereafter (reducing the risk of thromboembolism to 0.8%), unless the condition is known to be of short duration. Sotalol, flecainide and amiodarone reduce the risk of relapse after successful cardioversion. Nevertheless, at 1 month, 50% of patients will have reverted to atrial fibrillation. There is some evidence, however, that after subsequent attempts at defibrillation, sinus rhythm tends to become more stable and the interval between relapses increases.

Basic science

The heart rate is controlled under normal circumstances by rhythmic discharge from the sinoatrial node in the right atrial wall. This is controlled by the sympathetic and parasympathetic supply to the heart and by circulating levels of epinephrine, which between them set the rate to between 45 and 180 b.p.m. Parasympathetic tone is mediated by the vagus nerve which originates from the medulla oblongata. Sympathetic input is derived from the spinal cord at the T2 to T4 level. Other factors, such as blood temperature, pH, ionic composition and the concentrations of other hormones such as thyroxine, have a significant but smaller influence on the heart rate. Changes in heart rate and inotropic activity ensure that the blood pressure remains relatively constant despite rapid and dramatic changes in peripheral tissue oxygen demand.

MCQs

1 The incidence of atrial fibrillation increases with age.
2 Atrial fibrillation is associated with mitral stenosis and hypothyroidism.
3 The onset of atrial fibrillation is associated with a 30% reduction in cardiac output.
4 Warfarin treatment markedly reduces the thromboembolic risk of atrial fibrillation.
5 If untreated, acute atrial fibrillation is likely to revert spontaneously to sinus rhythm.

Case 18

High blood pressure and a family history

History

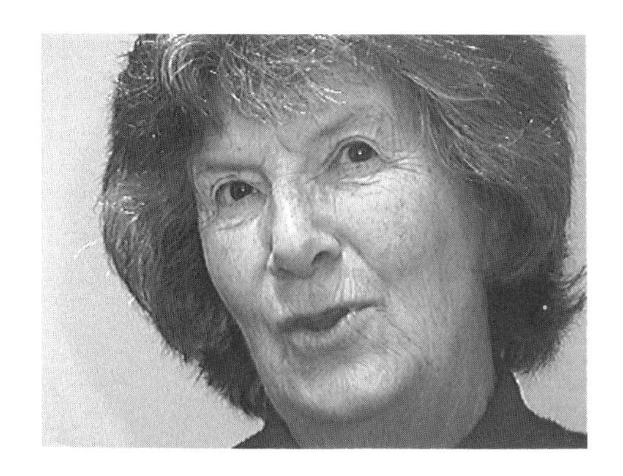

A 63-year-old housewife was seen in the renal clinic with hypertension and gradually progressive chronic renal failure that had first been diagnosed 13 years previously. Her mother had died of renal failure at the age of 54 years and her grandmother, it was thought, had died of the same condition also in middle age. The patient herself had tried to ignore the possibility that she had inherited a problem, but did know that she had high blood pressure and that this had been a feature of her mother's condition. During the preceding 18 months, her appetite had diminished, and she had noted an increasing number of episodes when she felt extremely tired and lethargic. She denied dysuria or polyuria at any time but, on one occasion, had passed blood in her urine. On examination, the principal finding was abdominal fullness without a fluid thrill or shifting dullness. Her blood pressure was 154/98 mmHg.

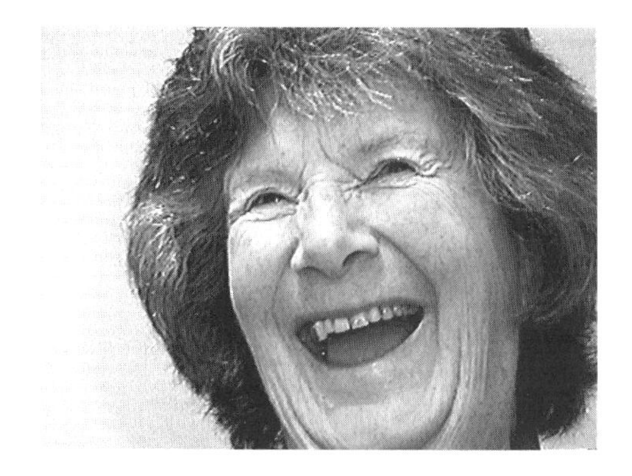

Notes

The patient presented with the symptoms and signs of chronic renal failure which, in her case, was secondary to polycystic renal disease.

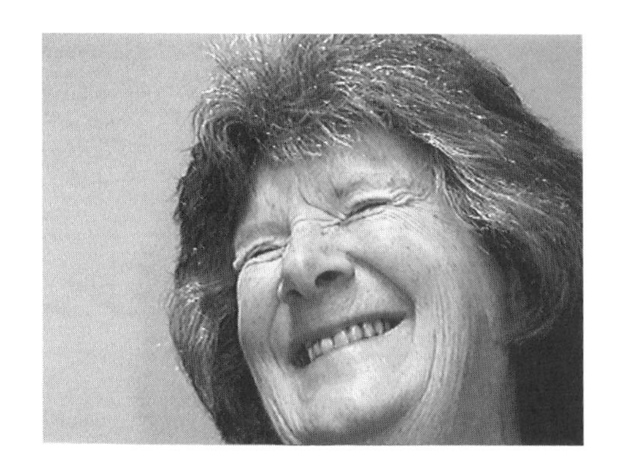

Two of her three children were also affected by polycystic renal disease, which is an autosomal dominant condition responsible for around 10% of cases of end-stage chronic renal failure that affects 0.1% of the population. Most cases of autosomal dominant polycystic renal disease are associated with mutations of polycystin-1 and polycystin-2, the products of the *PKD1* and *PKD2* genes. The cortex and medulla of the kidneys fill with thin-walled cysts up to several centimetres in diameter that eventually cause marked enlargement of the kidneys and interfere with their function. Common symptoms are:

- haematuria,
- flank pain,
- palpably enlarged kidneys,
- failure to concentrate the urine,
- proteinuria, and
- a predisposition to calculi formation.

When chronic renal failure supervenes, drowsiness and malaise, itching and neuromuscular complications, such as restless legs (jumpy legs particularly at night), are relatively common. Hepatic cysts are present in 30% of patients, but hepatic function is usually preserved, and patients tend not to be as anaemic as other patients with chronic (untreated) renal impairment. Subarachnoid haemorrhage from intracranial aneurysms is the cause of death in 9% of patients with polycystic renal disease.

Basic science

Chronic renal failure

Chronic renal failure is the result of sustained, progressive renal injury that, despite successful treatment of predisposing factors, such as hypertension, urinary tract obstruction or infection and systemic diseases (such as vasculitis), inexorably destroys nephron mass. The most common cause is glomerulonephritis, and the most common cause of that is immunoglobulin A (IgA) disease (see below). The consequences of chronic renal failure are the retention of products of metabolism such as urea, and the failure of the various metabolic and endocrine functions of the kidney. The reciprocal creatinine plot (reciprocal serum creatinine against time) predicts terminal renal failure and the requirement for dialysis.

Volume and electrolyte problems occur almost invariably and, although there is relative cellular hypokalaemia, serum potassium levels and potassium loss into the stools are usually high, owing to acidosis and insulin resistance (insulin facilitates the cellular uptake of potassium ions). Hypertriglyceridaemia and, to a lesser extent, hypercholesterolaemia are common in chronic renal failure, and contribute to accelerated atherosclerosis in these patients.

Renal osteodystrophy is the result of decreased activation of vitamin D (which impairs calcium absorption from the gut), retention of toxic metabolites, protein-calorie malnutrition, which impairs bone growth, and hyperphosphataemia leading to reciprocal hypocalcaemia and hyperparathyroidism. Severe acidosis is treated with sodium bicarbonate or citrate, and calcium and activated vitamin D (1α-hydroxycholecalciferol) supplements are given to reduce parathyroid hormone levels. Normochromic, normocytic anaemia, caused by failure of erythropoietin production, can be corrected (to some extent at the expense of blood pressure control) by injections of recombinant human erythropoietins. Careful dietary protein restriction can also slow the progression of chronic renal failure.

As the kidneys are responsible for polypeptide hormone metabolism, circulating levels of parathyroid hormone, insulin, prolactin, growth hormone and other hormones tend to rise.

IgA nephropathy (synonymous with mesangial IgA disease and Berger's disease) is the most common pattern of glomerulonephritis worldwide. The classification is based on the histological identification of mesangial deposits of IgA, and can be made without any histological evidence of associated injury. Damage associated with IgA deposits varies from trivial glomerular hypercellularity to advanced glomerular sclerosis, tubular atrophy and interstitial fibrosis coupled with renal failure. Clinically, episodes of macroscopic haematuria provoked by urinary tract infections are common in children and young adults with IgA disease. Microscopic haematuria is almost universal in IgA disease, and presentation with chronic renal impairment, proteinuria and hypertension is common. End-stage renal disease develops slowly and affects around 25% of patients at 25 years.

The renal involvement in Henoch–Schönlein purpura is almost identical in nature, and has led to the concept that Henoch–Schönlein purpura and IgA nephropathy are two manifestations of the same condition.

MCQs

1 Polycystic renal disease causes 25% of cases of end-stage chronic renal failure.
2 Polycystic renal disease is associated with intracranial aneurysms.
3 Hepatic cysts in polycystic renal disease can lead to cirrhosis in dialysed patients.
4 In chronic renal failure, the reciprocal creatinine plot can be used to predict time to end-stage renal failure.
5 Special dietary restrictions can slow the progression of chronic renal failure.

Case 19
Intermittent loin pain: the ping in the pan

History

A 67-year-old paper bag printer was seen in clinic with a history of recurrent episodes of very severe pain radiating from the right inguinal region to the tip of his penis. The pain came on initially during the day, but subsequently occurred at any time of the day or night, and lasted for several hours or days at a time. The pain was constant in nature rather than colicky, and was associated with sweating. The patient denied any change in his bowel or urinary habit, and there was no history of haematuria. There were no exacerbating or relieving factors and, on examination, no intra-abdominal or genitourinary abnormality could be detected. At the time of examination, the patient was not tender to percussion over the flanks. A plain abdominal radiograph revealed a small opacity overlying the lower end of the right ureter. Over a period of several months, during which the patient experienced repeated attacks of abdominal pain which eventually gave way to almost constant pain, the stone remained static within the ureter. In the anteroom of the operating room, the patient was asked if he would try to empty his bladder and, when he did so, he heard a 'ping' and noticed a fragment the size of his little fingernail in the pan.

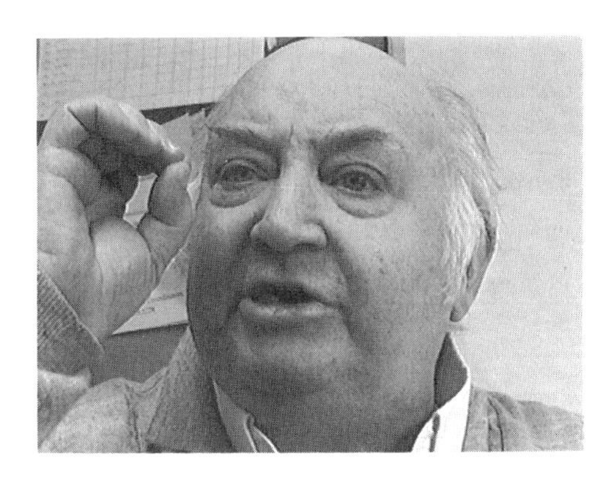

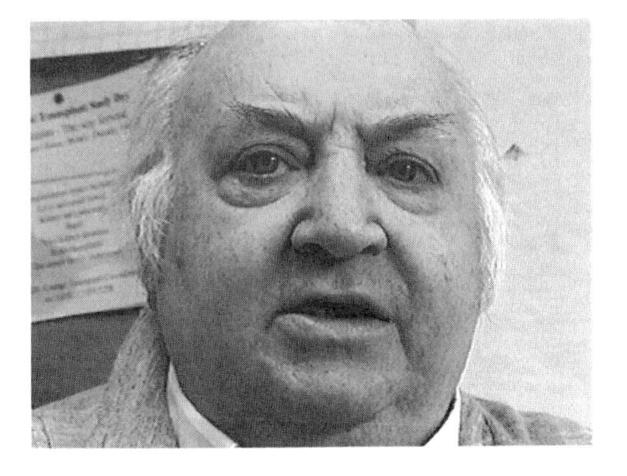

Notes

The patient had renal stones and suffered repeated attacks of renal colic.

Asymptomatic stones are often discovered incidentally on abdominal X-rays taken for other reasons, or during investigation for microscopic or macroscopic haematuria. If the stones block the junction of the renal pelvis with the ureter, or migrate down into the ureter itself, severe flank pain rising to a peak over 20–60 min and bleeding often result. Pain that migrates down into the loin, testis or vulva indicates that the stone has moved into the lower third of the ureter, and impaction of the stone within the ureter that traverses the bladder wall can produce symptoms reminiscent of a urinary tract infection. Indications for stone removal are:

- inferction,
- obstruction,
- bleeding, and
- severe pain.

Basic science

Renal stone formation

Almost all renal stones are formed from a mixture of calcium salts (usually calcium oxalate or calcium phosphate, which account for 80% of stones), uric acid (radiolucent stones which account for 5–8%) or struvite (magnesium ammonium phosphate). Young men are most commonly affected, and the tendency to stone formation, which is familial, does not wane with time. Struvite stones, the second commonest type (10–15%), are precipitated mostly in women by urinary tract infections with urease-producing bacteria, and give rise to 'staghorn' calculi that may fill the renal pelvis and calyces.

Other factors that predispose to nephrolithiasis include hereditary distal renal tubular acidosis, urinary supersaturation with uric acid or cystine, either due to their overproduction or decreased urine volume (such as dehydration), and causes of hypercalciuria, such as hypoparathyroidism, particularly with excessive calcium and vitamin D therapy, or idiopathic hypercalciuria.

In some patients with idiopathic hypercalciuria, gastrointestinal absorption of calcium is excessive and the rise in calcium causes postprandial suppression of parathyroid hormone secretion. Renal tubular absorption of calcium is decreased and the calcium saturation of the filtrate increases. In others, the primary problem seems to be decreased renal tubular reabsorption of calcium.

MCQs

1 Eighty per cent of renal stones are made predominantly of calcium oxalate and calcium phosphate.
2 Renal stones invariably produce symptoms of renal colic.
3 Staghorn calculi are usually made of calcium oxalate.
4 The tendency to stone formation tends to decrease with time.
5 Causes of hypercalcaemia are associated with increased renal stone formation.

Case 20
Breathlessness and a productive cough

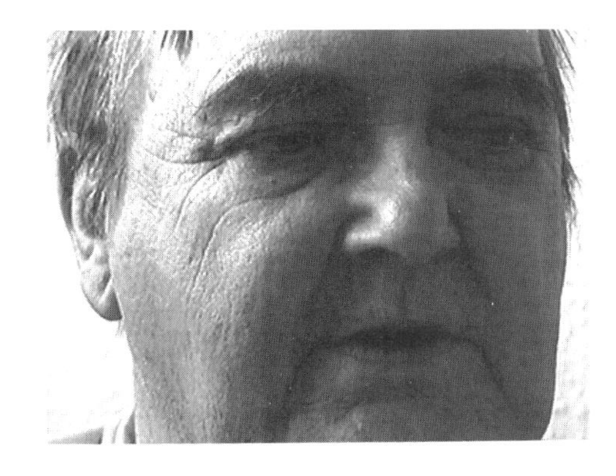

History

A 63-year-old former lighthouse keeper, who had smoked 20–30 cigarettes daily since the age of 15 years, was admitted to hospital with an exacerbation of shortness of breath and cough. He had suffered from a cough for as long as he could remember, but did not have any exercise limitation until 9 years previously when he suffered a myocardial infarction. From that time on, his exercise capacity became gradually more limited, and his admissions to hospital with infective exacerbations of his airways' disease became more frequent. For the 6 months prior to his admission, he was able to walk only 25 paces without stopping, was unable to ascend stairs and was using oxygen at home continuously. He also complained that his sleeping at night was disturbed, but that he tended to nod off during the day.

On examination, his chest was mildly hyperexpanded, and crackles and coarse breath sounds were noted throughout all fields. His core temperature was 37.2 °C, but his sputum was purulent. Blood cultures were negative.

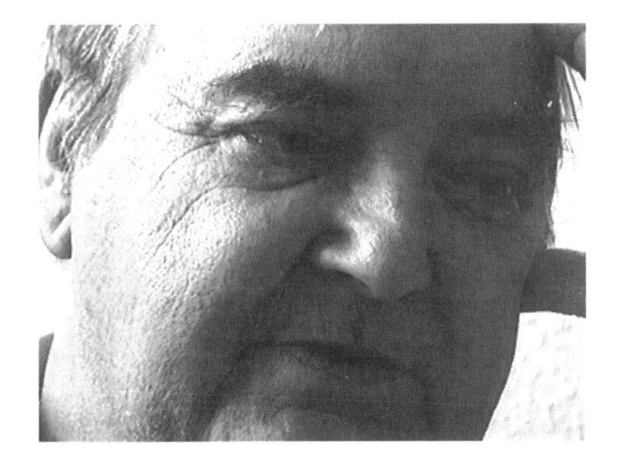

Notes

The patient had an infective exacerbation of chronic obstructive pulmonary disease.

Chronic obstructive pulmonary disease is a slowly progressive airways' disorder that remains fairly stable over time, although punctuated by infective exacerbations characterized by increased purulent sputum production. It usually has a minimal reversible component, with no significant response to oral steroids. The patients have typically smoked a packet of cigarettes daily for 20 years or more, and experience chronic, pro-

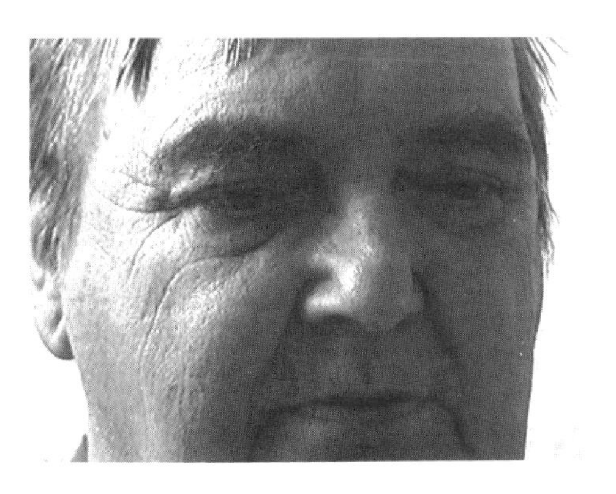

gressive breathlessness with little variability accompanied by evidence of airflow obstruction on lung function testing. Obstruction to expiratory airflow (reduction in the forced expiratory volume in 1 s, FEV1) is present and, to a large extent, fixed. Further progressive decline in lung function leads eventually to death by respiratory or cardiorespiratory failure. When the FEV1 is less than 40% of predicted, the condition is classified as severe, and the 5-year survival is less than 50%.

Basic science

Epidemiology of smoking-related disease

Smoking-related deaths are currently running at around 3 000 000 annually worldwide, and are set to increase over threefold during the next 40 years. More than half of all smokers die of smoking-related diseases. Lung cancer kills 7% of males who smoke, and is now more common a cause of death in females than breast cancer. Smoking is the most important cause of chronic obstructive pulmonary disease and, amongst male smokers aged over 65 years, about one-quarter have symptoms suggestive of chronic obstructive pulmonary disease. The cough eventually ceases if sufferers stop smoking and, in most cases, the rate of decline in pulmonary function decreases to age-related control levels.

Chronic obstructive pulmonary disease

Chronic bronchitis, which often accompanies chronic obstructive pulmonary disease, is cough with expectoration for 3 months of each of two successive years which cannot be attributed to other pulmonary causes.

Emphysema is the permanent destructive enlargement of airways distal to terminal bronchioles without fibrosis. This can occur particularly rapidly when intrinsic enzyme systems that protect the lung from proteolytic enzymes, such as α_1-antitrypsin, are absent.

Asthma is an inflammatory disease of the airways, producing limitation to expiratory airflow that characteristically improves with glucocorticoid treatment.

The FEV1 is a useful measure in chronic obstructive pulmonary disease, because the method is standardized, the test is reproducible and the normal ranges for age and sex are very well defined. When the FEV1/FVC ratio (FVC, forced vital capacity) is less than 70% and the FEV1 is less than 80% of that predicted for age, the FEV1 predicts both the degree of disability and the prognosis. The FEV1 can also be used to estimate the

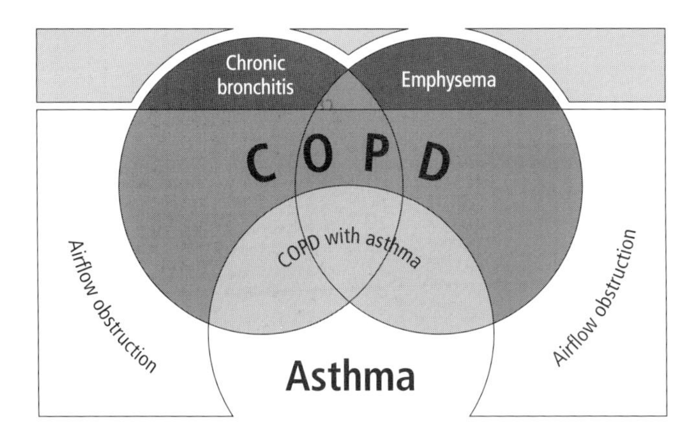

reversibility of the airflow obstruction, as an improvement of 15% or 200 mL suggests an element of bronchospasm (asthma).

Carbon dioxide retention

The principal effects of hypercapnia are on the central nervous system. Acute hypercapnia or the abrupt worsening of chronic hypercapnia—which, in itself, can be almost asymptomatic—produces cerebral vasodilatation, increased cerebrospinal fluid pressure, weakness, irritability and drowsiness, progressing to somnolence, confusion and coma. Carbon dioxide retention is a self-perpetuating event as it depresses the response of the respiratory centre to hypoxia. Patients are thus particularly sensitive to the central nervous system depressant effects of sedatives, or to the abolition of peripheral respiratory drive by breathing supplemental oxygen. Carbon dioxide retention leads to acidosis which is compensated by bicarbonate retention by the kidneys.

MCQs

1 Second to breast cancer, lung cancer is the most common cause of neoplastic death in women.
2 Patients with chronic obstructive pulmonary disease usually show marked variability in lung function over time.
3 When the FEV1 is less than 40% of predicted, the 5-year survival is less than 50%.
4 About 25% of smokers die of smoking-related disease.
5 The FEV1 is a useful measure of the reversibility of airflow obstruction.

Case 21
Chest pain and breathlessness

History

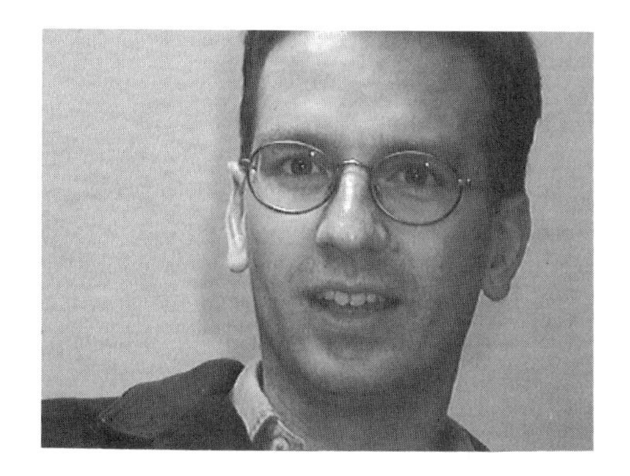

A 29-year-old businessman woke up to find that he had some discomfort on the right side of his chest. Initially, he assumed that he had slept awkwardly and took little notice of the pain. However, the discomfort worsened during the day and began to be associated with shortness of breath. He presented to the local accident and emergency department and explained that he had no previous history of chest infection or cough, could not recollect injuring or straining himself in any way and had been perfectly well the night before. On examination, he looked well, but was clearly anxious about the pain. Percussion of his chest was resonant, and breath sounds appeared to be normal bilaterally. Although no difference could be detected between the two sides of his chest, his trachea was noted to be displaced to the left and he was mildly tachypnoeic. An ECG was normal. A **chest X-ray** revealed the diagnosis.

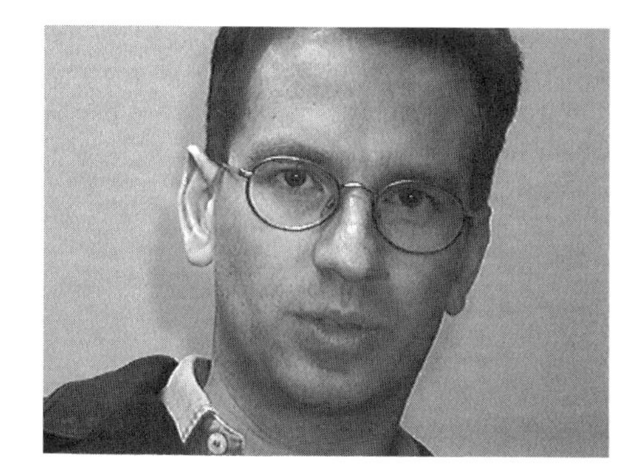

Notes

The patient had suffered a spontaneous pneumothorax.

A pneumothorax is a collection of air in the pleural space that arises either from a communication of the pleural cavity with the skin or the airways, in association with partial or, as was the case here, complete collapse of the lung. The pressure in the pleural cavity is usually negative with respect to the atmosphere, and it is this that holds the lungs inflated inside the pleural cavity. If the pressure in the pleural cavity matches atmospheric pressure, the elastic recoil of the lungs makes them collapse, and, if the pressure exceeds atmospheric (which occurs when the air leak into the pleural cavity assumes a valve-like

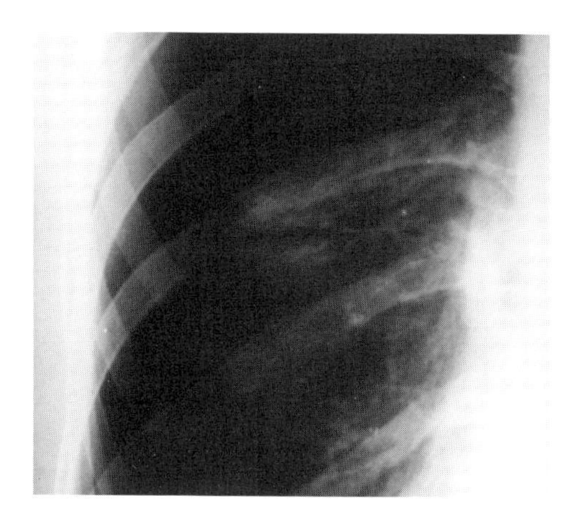

action), the mediastinum is displaced to the opposite side (tension pneumothorax) and heart function can be compromised. Tension pneumothorax is a medical emergency.

Basic science

Causes of pneumothorax

Previously healthy, thin adults between the ages of 20 and 40 years are most susceptible to spontaneous and sometimes recurrent pneumothoraces, caused in many cases by rupture of small blebs on the apical surface of the lungs. In patients over 40 years of age, spontaneous pneumothorax is most often associated with *chronic obstructive pulmonary disease*, in which progressive destruction of alveolar walls is associated with intermittent high intrapulmonary pressures caused by coughing. *Asthma* may also be associated with the development of pneumothorax and, in the past, *rupture of cavities*, such as caseating subpleural tuberculosis, staphylococcal pneumonia or bronchogenic carcinoma, were significant causes. *Industrial lung diseases*, such as coal miners' pneumoconiosis, silicosis and exposure to beryllium and, particularly, aluminium dust, are also implicated.

Pleura

The visceral and parietal pleurae (covering the lungs and the chest wall, respectively), derived from the splanchnic and parietal mesoderm lining the pericardioperitoneal canal, constitute a continuous membrane that contains a small amount of fluid under negative pressure. The fluid is a filtrate produced by the parietal pleura and resorbed by the visceral pleura. Changes in hydrostatic or osmotic pressure in heart failure, hepatic failure or renal failure, for example, lead to the formation of a low protein pleural transudate (<30 g protein L^{-1}). Changes in the permeability of the pleura that occur in inflammatory or neoplastic processes result in the formation of a high protein pleural exudate. Activation of the sensory innervation of the pleural membranes gives rise to sharp, localized pain exacerbated by inspiration; irritation of the diaphragmatic pleura gives rise to pain referred to the shoulder. The result is shallow, rapid breathing with reduced diaphragmatic movements, particularly on the affected side. Auscultation often reveals a pleural friction rub that can be heard almost throughout the respiratory cycle.

MCQs

1 At the end of normal expiration, intrathoracic pressure matches atmospheric pressure.
2 The pleura, like the lungs, is endodermal in origin.
3 Irritation of the diaphragmatic pleura leads to pain referred to the shoulder.
4 Pleural fluid is a filtrate produced by the parietal pleura.
5 Inflammation of the pleura typically gives rise to a poorly localized, aching pain.

Case 22
Cough, malaise and chest pain

History

A 35-year-old physiotherapist and mother of three was admitted to hospital with a 9-day history of a non-productive cough exacerbated by lying down, associated with lethargy, malaise and aching muscles, particularly the shoulder girdle. This had been accompanied by fevers and chills, anorexia and insomnia and, on one occasion, after a particularly strenuous coughing bout, some sharp chest pain. She had received all of her childhood immunizations, including BCG (bacillus Calmette–Guérin) vaccine at the age of 13 years, and had undergone two subsequent tuberculin tests, all of which to her knowledge showed that she was immune to tuberculosis. After 2 days of treatment with antibiotics from her doctor, she felt worse and, on review, was referred to hospital. She denied any contacts with people known to have chest infections, and had not been abroad.

On examination, the patient was anxious and very lethargic. Her temperature fluctuated from 37 °C to 38.4 °C during the course of her first inpatient day. No lymphadenopathy was present. She was noted to be slightly tachypnoeic, and was dull to percussion at the left base. Crackles were heard throughout her left lung field, with bronchial breathing in the mid and upper zones.

A **chest X-ray** showed basal consolidation on the left with a further area of loss of transradiance in the upper zone, together with air bronchograms. Sputum was initially not available for culture, but her blood cultures and urine cultures were negative.

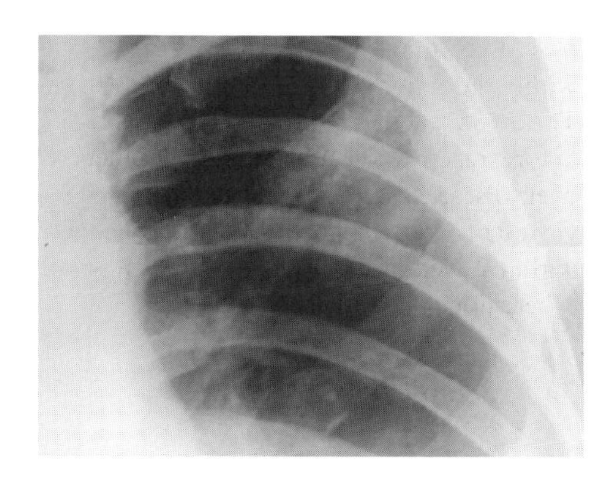

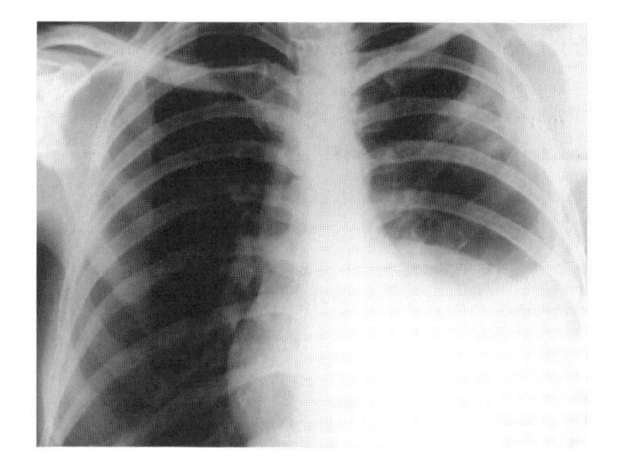

Notes

The patient had pulmonary tuberculosis. A sputum sample revealed the presence of acid-fast bacilli on Ziehl–Nielsen staining. Subsequent culture was positive for *Mycobacterium tuberculosis*.

Tuberculosis is a chronic bacterial infection caused by *Mycobacterium tuberculosis*. The surface lipids on mycobacteria prevent them from being decolorized after staining by immersion in acid alcohol. Hence their description as 'acid fast'. The usual route of infection is by inhalation and as few as 1–3 airborne desiccated *M. tuberculosis* organisms derived from the respiratory secretions of an infected individual are sufficient to cause disease. The usual site of primary infection is the lung. Caseating granuloma, the characteristic histology of *M. tuberculosis*, is the result of the highly antigenic nature of the organism, its ability to remain intact after phagocytosis by macrophages and the florid cell-mediated hypersensitivity that is induced. In at least 95% of cases, the mild, non-specific inflammation of the primary infection is fully contained within the regional lymph nodes and heals up. The organism may lie dormant for many years before reactivation and the development of overt disease.

Patients are usually rendered non-infectious within 2 weeks of the start of effective antituberculous chemotherapy.

Basic science

Infectious organisms

To qualify as infectious, an organism has to be able to remain alive until it enters the host, and then either avoid or survive phagocytosis and highly toxic oxygen intermediates produced by the host's local respiratory bursts, while finding sufficient nutrients to grow and reproduce. The infectious organism then has to compete with commensal organisms and with its own progeny or the progeny of adjacent organisms whilst, at least in some circumstances, maintaining transcription of whatever plasmids confer antibiotic resistance for the subsequent iatrogenic onslaught.

Bacteria. Bacteria are free-living, unicellular prokaryotes that typically cause wound, urinary and gastrointestinal infections. They can grow extracellularly or intracellularly and produce endo- or exotoxins. They have very high rates of protein synthesis that allow them to divide during exponential growth every 20 min. Many types of bacteria are also able to take up DNA fragments from other strains of bacteria when lysed. It is salutary to remember that 80% of the entire history of evolution took place within unicellular organisms.

Viruses. Viruses are obligate intracellular parasites with relatively simple genomes encoded in either DNA or ribonucleic acid (RNA). They exploit the protein and DNA/RNA synthetic apparatus of the host cell and are often directly cytopathogenic. Some viruses have the capacity for latency, and in the case of herpes zoster, for example, can remain within specific sites, such as the posterior root ganglia, for decades before reactivation.

Fungi. Fungi are free-living uni- or multicellular organisms that are frequently opportunistic or saprophytic. They form extensive hyphal networks or exist in yeast-like forms.

Protozoa. Protozoa are free-living unicellular eukaryotes, such as *Plasmodium* sp. (malaria), *Entamoeba histolytica* (amoebic dysentery or liver abscesses) or *Trypanosoma cruzi*, that have complex life cycles often involving multiple host species and insect vectors. *Plasmodium*, *Toxoplasma* and *Trypanosoma* are examples of obligate intracellular parasites. *Entamoeba histolytica* are free-living organisms.

Helminths. The nematodes (roundworms), trematodes (flatworms) and cestodes (tapeworms), such as *Ascaris lumbricoides*, *Schistosoma mansoni* and *Taenia solium*, are intestinal, blood and lymphatic parasites with complex life cycles involving multiple host species.

Prions. Prions are infectious proteins implicated in scrapie in sheep, bovine spongiform encephalopathy and the human variant of the same. They appear to function by inducing abnormal folding of target proteins which then influence other proteins to 'misfold' in the same way.

MCQs

1 The hypoxaemia of pneumonia results from shunting of the blood away from the affected lung.
2 In pneumonia, the compliance of the lung and tidal volumes tend to decrease.

3 Cytomegalovirus is a typical cause of pneumonia in immunocompromised hosts.
4 The infective dose of *Mycobacterium tuberculosis* can be as little as a single organism.
5 Patients with open tuberculosis are typically still infectious 2 months after the start of chemotherapy.

Case 23
Haemoptysis and a pain in the neck

History

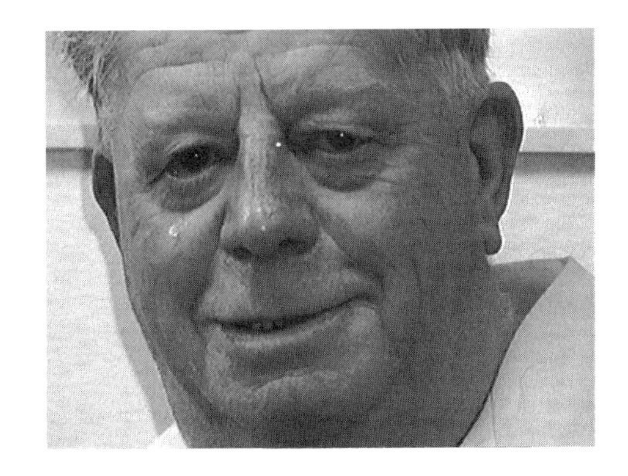

A 74-year-old retired civil servant presented with a 3-week history of haemoptysis. He had a history of mild shortness of breath on exertion and a cough that he had ascribed to smoking and taken little notice of. To his alarm, for 3 weeks leading up to his admission, his sputum had been deeply blood-stained and, on some occasions, appeared to consist almost entirely of blood. This had been accompanied by swelling and discomfort on the right side of his neck that were worse in the morning, but not with any chest pain or worsening of his breathlessness. He had a past history of an appendicectomy, and had undergone two operations on his testes for torsion and hydrocoele. In Italy, during the Second World War, he sustained major injuries to his right lung in a mortar attack while mine sweeping, but recovered well.

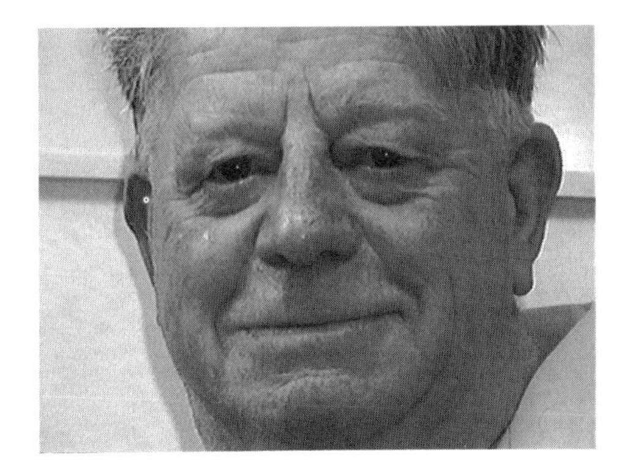

On examination, he was anxious but apyrexial. Breath sounds were reduced bilaterally and replaced, particularly over the right mid and upper zones, with crackles and a fixed wheeze. His neck was tender to palpation, but no discrete or diffuse masses were palpable.

Notes

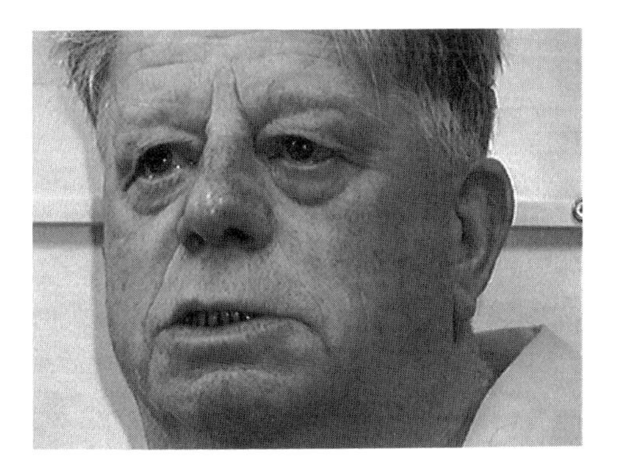

The patient had developed a bronchogenic neoplasm.

With the exception of chest pain, this patient experienced all of the important symptoms of respiratory disease, namely cough, sputum production, breathlessness, wheeze and **haemoptysis**. Smoking-induced chronic obstructive pulmonary disease further reduced the fixed airflow limitation resulting from traumatic damage to the right lung. Smoking was also responsible for increasing his risk of developing bronchogenic carcinoma. The cause of his intermittent neck pain and swelling was unclear, as there was no confirmatory evidence of superior vena cava obstruction, lymph node or nerve involvement at presentation.

Chronic obstructive pulmonary disease, which encompasses the terms 'chronic bronchitis' and 'emphysema' and the 'blue bloater' and 'pink puffer' phenotypes, is characterized by airflow obstruction, particularly on expiration, that ultimately leads to respiratory or cardiorespiratory failure. The condition is closely related to the history of tobacco smoking in most patients. The characteristic feature of the condition is a steady, but abnormally rapid, age-related, non-reversible decline in the forced expiratory volume in 1 s (FEV1) that is independent of the hypersecretion of mucus, cough or sputum production. As the changes are irreversible and largely beyond pharmacotherapy, management is difficult and the best approach is prevention.

There is no pathological distinction between the 'blue bloater' and 'pink puffer' phenotypes, but they may reflect different patterns of ventilatory control and require different clinical management.

Basic science

Aetiology of haemoptysis

- Bronchogenic carcinoma.
- Chest infections:
  - Tuberculosis.
  - Lobar pneumonia (typically pneumococcal, staphylococcal, *Klebsiella pneumoniae*).
- Pulmonary embolism with pulmonary infarction.
- Bronchiectasis.
- Aspergilloma within a cavity.
- Chronic obstructive pulmonary disease.
- Foreign body.
- Vasculitis:
  - Wegener's granulomatosis.
  - Goodpastures.
  - Polyarteritis nodosa.
- Hereditary haemorrhagic telangiectasia.
- Mitral stenosis or pulmonary oedema.

Smoking

Cigarette smoke is a complex mixture of more than 4000 substances, some of which have pharmacological, cytotoxic and mutagenic activity. The principal pharmacological effects of cigarette smoke are mediated by nicotine (a toxic, addictive and cardioactive alkaloid), aromatic hydrocarbons, amines and nitrosamines that form a carcinogenic condensate, and carbon monoxide. Carbon monoxide interferes with oxygen transport and utilization, and reaches concentrations as high as 6% in cigarette smoke. Carboxyhaemoglobin levels, normally around 1%, are fivefold higher in smokers than in non-smokers.

Cigarette smokers have a 70% higher death rate than non-smokers. In 35-year-old men who smoke, the risks of dying before the age of 65 years increase almost threefold compared with non-smokers. Men who smoke 20 cigarettes daily increase their risk of dying from lung cancer by 10-fold. Men who smoke 40 cigarettes daily increase their risks by 25-fold. The risk of dying from chronic obstructive pulmonary disease is also strongly related to cigarette smoking, increasing from fourfold to 25-fold, and all outcomes of pregnancy are adversely affected.

Dust diseases

Occupational lung diseases are the result of damage to the lungs caused by the inhalation of dusts (aerosols composed of solid inert particles; pneumoconiosis caused by coal dust, kaolin (china clay), talc, silica and asbestos), fumes (such as ammonia, chlorine, sulphur dioxide) or other noxious substances, such as irritants and organic dusts (for example byssinosis, bagassosis and farmer's lung, caused by the inhalation of cotton dust, sugar cane dust or thermophilic actinomycete spores (affecting 1–5% of farmers), respectively). The most prevalent of the pneumoconioses are coal miners' pneumoconiosis (affecting 12% of all coal miners and up to 50% of anthracite miners), caused by prolonged exposure to coal dust particles of about 5 μm in diameter (large enough to be carried into the alveoli, but too large to remain suspended), and silicosis (exposure to free crystalline quartz (SiO_2) or the less hazardous silicates, such as kaolin, mica, cement dusts, etc., where the risk is related to the free silica content) in mining, quarrying and fettling (grinding metal fillets off castings).

Free dust particles and dust-laden macrophages lead to fibrosis. Progressive massive fibrosis leads to round fibrotic masses of several centimetres in diameter in the upper lobes.

An excess risk of lung squamous cell carcinoma or adenocarcinoma is associated with asbestos exposure after a latent period of 15–19 years. Concurrent cigarette smoking produces a synergistic mutagenic effect, and the more intense the exposure to asbestos, the greater the risk.

Mesotheliomas are also associated with asbestos exposure, the risk peaking up to 35 years after initial exposure. The risk is not amplified by concurrent smoking.

MCQs

1 The 'pink puffer' and 'blue bloater' phenotypes of chronic obstructive pulmonary disease can be distinguished by histological examination of the lungs.
2 Coal miners' pneumoconiosis is caused by inhalation of coal dust particles of 5 μm in diameter.
3 The risk of lung cancer increases within 10 years of asbestos exposure.
4 Exposure to asbestos and smoking have an additive effect on lung cancer risk.
5 Between 1 and 5% of farmers suffer from occupational lung disease.

Case 24
Sudden onset of shortness of breath

History

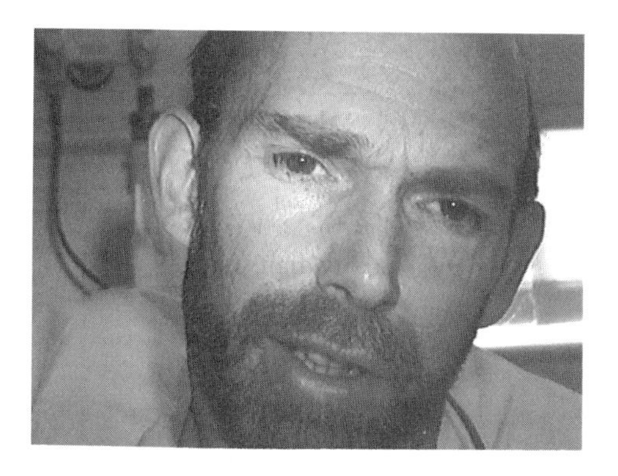

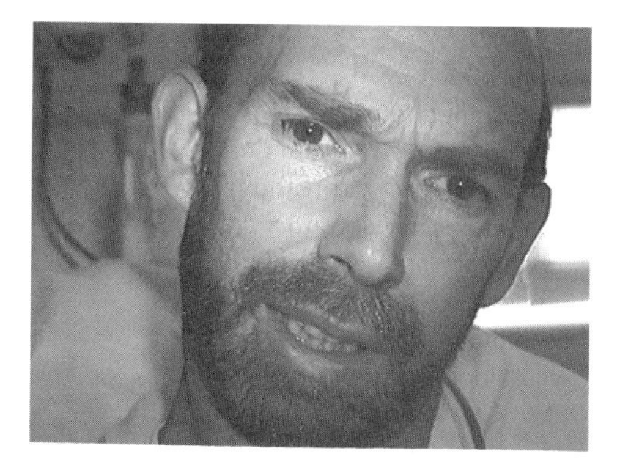

A 43-year-old teacher was admitted to accident and emergency with a 3-h history of rapidly increasing breathlessness and wheeze. Since the age of 16 years, he had suffered from asthma and, despite prophylactic treatment, had become used to 'being slightly tight' almost every morning. Breathing in cold air tended to exacerbate his tendency to wheeze, but there were no other acute exacerbating or relieving factors, no seasonal effects and he had no specific allergies as far as he knew. At the time of admission, his only treatment was salbutamol by inhalation as required.

On examination, the patient was sitting up on the edge of the bed, anxious and sweating with a respiratory rate of $30\,min^{-1}$. A loud wheeze was heard on auscultation of all areas of his chest, and his systolic blood pressure varied from 180 mmHg on expiration to 126 mmHg during inspiration. A chest X-ray was hyperexpanded, but did not show any evidence of infection or pneumothorax.

Notes

The patient was suffering an **acute asthma attack**.

Asthma is produced by widespread, episodic narrowing of the airways in response to a wide range of stimuli lasting minutes or hours, causing wheezing, dyspnoea and cough. The patient often recovers completely between attacks. Respiratory infections, emotional stress and exercise, particularly when the temperature of the inspired air is low, are the most common provocative stimuli to asthma.

Allergic asthma is often associated with a personal or family history of rhinitis, urticaria and eczema, a positive response to provocative tests and a raised immunoglobulin E (IgE). Inhalation of very small quantities of specific antigens induces lung mast cell degranulation with the release of bioactive peptides, such as histamine, bradykinin, leukotrienes, prostaglandins and thromboxane. These induce bronchospasm, increase the permeability of bronchial capillaries and stimulate migration of eosinophils and neutrophils to the site of degranulation.

Geographical and meteorological phenomena leading to stagnant air masses, heavy industrial activity and dense urbanization result in a build up of polluting antigens in the air that predispose susceptible people to asthma. Exposure to platinum, chromium and nickel salts in refining and plating, and to organic dusts, such as flour, grain, gums, coffee beans and sawdust, is associated with asthma. Industrial chemicals, such as solvents and plastics, laundry detergents, animal dander and insect dusts can also precipitate acute attacks of bronchospasm.

Pathophysiology of asthma

The pathological changes of asthma are:

1 reduction in airway diameter;

2 oedema of the bronchial walls; and

3 the production of thick, tenacious secretions.

During an attack, there is:

- increased airway resistance,
- decreased forced expiratory volumes (≤ 50% of normal) and flow rates (the forced expiratory volume in 1 s, FEV1, averages 30% of predicted),
- hyperinflation of the lungs (residual volume increased fourfold) and thorax,
- increased work of breathing,
- alterations in respiratory muscle function,
- changes in elastic recoil,
- abnormal distribution of both ventilation and pulmonary blood flow and altered arterial blood gases.

The ECG often shows evidence of right ventricular hypertrophy and pulmonary hypertension.

Patients report that they feel normal after an attack of asthma when the functional residual capacity (the amount of air remaining in the lungs after a normal—rather than maximal—expiratory effort) is still double normal and the FEV1 is ≥50% of normal. Hypoxia is universal during an acute asthmatic attack, but ventilatory failure (normal or raised $P\mathrm{CO_2}$) is present in only 10–15% of patients admitted to hospital. Most asthmatics have a low $P\mathrm{CO_2}$ and respiratory alkalosis.

Basic science

Blood gas analysis

Carbon dioxide saturation. The principal acid product of metabolism is carbon dioxide. Its normal concentration in body fluids is 1.2 mmol L^{-1} (equivalent to a partial pressure of 5.3 kPa or 40 mmHg), at which level production matches pulmonary excretion. The $P_a\mathrm{CO_2}$ reflects the adequacy of volume of ventilation. A marked rise in CO_2 leads to tachycardia, a rise in blood pressure with a bounding pulse, sweating and warm extremities, muscle twitching, coarse tremor and increased intracranial pressure with papilloedema, headaches, confusion and coma.

Oxygen saturation. Reduced arterial O_2 saturation at sea level is caused by:

- the mismatch of ventilation and pulmonary blood flow (i.e. large amounts of pulmonary artery blood bypassing ventilated lung),
- intrapulmonary shunts (direct flow of pulmonary arterial blood into the pulmonary venous system),
- inadequate alveolar ventilation (poor respiratory effort), or
- impaired diffusion of O_2 from alveolar gas into the bloodstream.

When one-third or more of mixed venous blood passes underventilated lung, the arterial oxygen saturation will be reduced to below 90%. A further reduction in mixed venous blood oxygen saturation caused by exercise will reduce $P_a\mathrm{O_2}$ and cyanosis will appear or worsen. If exercise does not worsen desaturation, hypoventilation rather than primary pulmonary disease is the likely cause, and, if breathing 30% (certainly 100%) oxygen does not rapidly restore $P_a\mathrm{O_2}$, a major right to left shunt is present.

Air travel with respiratory disease

In commercial aircraft flying at ~10 000 m (30 000 ft), cabin air is pressurized to an altitude equivalent of 8000 ft (2450 m). At this level, gases expand by 30% (the ears 'pop') and, as the partial pressure of oxygen falls, a healthy passenger will drop his/her arterial oxygen tension from 12 kPa (90 mmHg) to 8 kPa (60 mmHg). Because of the shape of the oxyhaemoglobin dissociation curve, arterial oxygen saturation falls by only 4–5%. Patients who are mildly hypoxaemic on the ground (for example with chronic obstructive pulmonary disease or bronchiectasis), however, may become profoundly hypoxaemic in the air.

If a patient is fit enough to walk 50 m on the flat without breathlessness and is able to breathe a 15% oxygen atmosphere (i.e. 100% nitrogen through a 40% ventimask) for 20 min without discomfort or a fall in oxygen saturation to less than 85%, the risk of flying will be relatively low.

Features of acute, severe asthma

- PEFR (peak expiratory flow rate) ≤50% predicted or best.
- Cannot complete sentences in one breath.
- Respirations ≥ 25 breaths per minute.
- Pulse >110 beats per minute.

Life-threatening features

- PEFR <33% predicted or best.
- Silent chest, cyanosis or feeble respiratory effort.
- Bradycardia or hypotension.
- Exhaustion, confusion or coma.

MCQs

1 Patients with life-threatening asthma may not be distressed.
2 Treatment of acute asthma includes the use of sedatives when the patient is distressed.
3 In normal people, oxygen saturation decreases by 33% when flying at 30 000 ft.
4 After an acute asthma attack, patients feel 'back to normal' before pulmonary changes completely resolve.
5 Hypoxaemia is unusual except in life-threatening asthma.

Case 25
The man who felt that he'd wasted his life

History

A 32-year-old former building surveyor was seen in the outpatient department for the assessment of chronic renal failure. He had been diagnosed with insulin-dependent diabetes at the age of 12 years, and remembered vividly being 'injected repeatedly in the leg with a large, blunt needle'. As his blood sugars remained high throughout his childhood and teenage years, he rarely suffered from hypoglycaemic episodes and, remaining essentially symptom free, considered himself 'a mild diabetic'. Three years previously he had suffered a detached retina on the right side with loss of most of the sight on that side. While waiting for surgery to reattach the retina, he had a vitreous haemorrhage on the left side and was rendered almost blind. His vision improved over several months to the extent that he could navigate around the shops, but he remained unable to manage entirely alone and could no longer enjoy watching television or reading. After remaining away from direct medical care for almost a year, he changed to a new GP and, at a routine medical, was found to have marked proteinuria. Routine biochemistry revealed a urea level of 15 $mmol\,L^{-1}$ (normal range = 3–7 $mmol\,L^{-1}$) and a creatinine level of 180 $\mu mol\,L^{-1}$ (normal range = $<120\,\mu mol\,L^{-1}$). On examination, he was able to detect finger movements only, but had no evidence of significant peripheral neuropathy. His blood pressure was 146/82 mmHg, and a 24-h collection of urine was found to contain 3 g of protein.

Notes

After years of poorly controlled diabetes mellitus, the patient had developed severe diabetic retinopathy and nephropathy.

The longer the duration of diabetes and the worse the control, the higher the prevalence and severity of retinopathy, neuropathy and nephropathy. Histological changes of diabetic nephropathy take at least 3 years to develop from biochemical diagnosis, and clinically significant proteinuria (in excess of 3–4 times normal) seldom occurs before the patient has had diabetes for 15 years. Microalbuminuria, urinary albumin excretion above normal but below the sensitivity of standard dipsticks, is a powerful predictor of diabetic nephropathy, end-stage renal disease, cardiovascular disease and premature death. Proteinuria at 0.5 g per day predicts end-stage renal failure or death

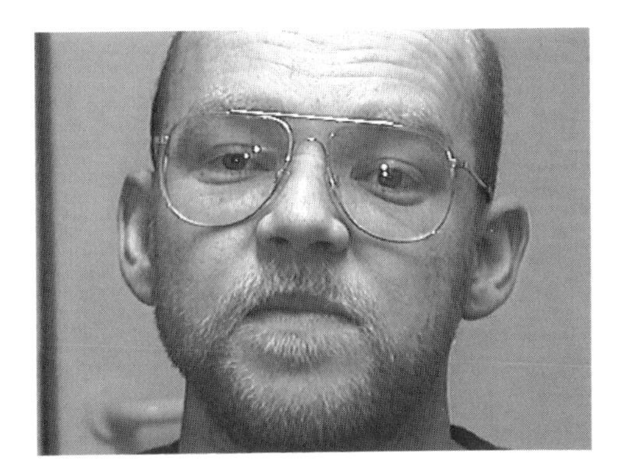

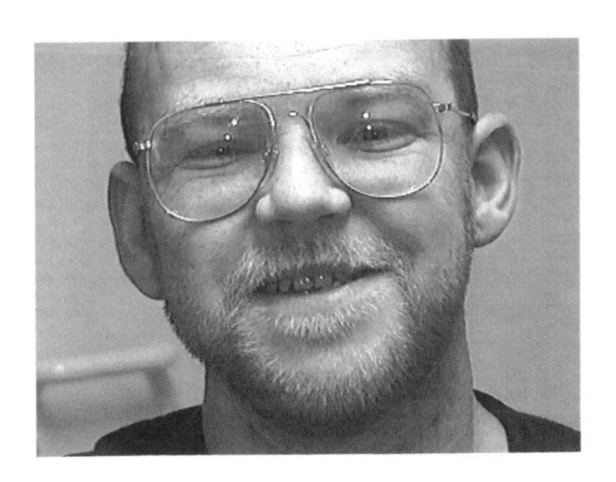

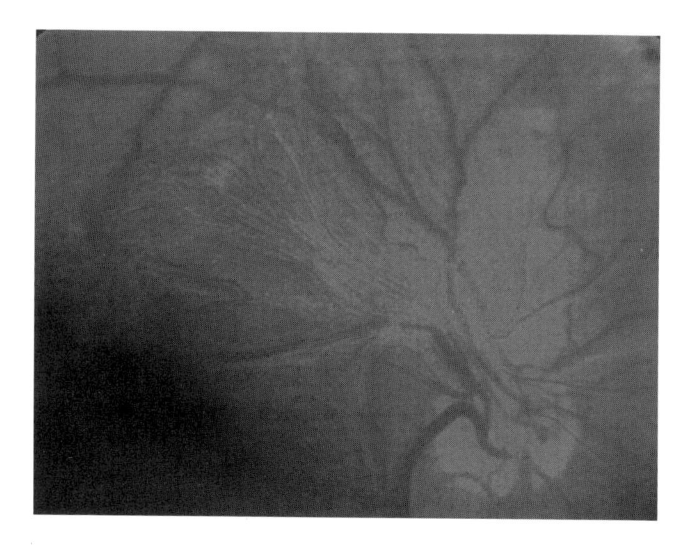

within 5 years and, when protein loss exceeds 5 g per day, mortality at 2 years (largely through the increased risk of coronary heart disease) is as high as 50%. Nephropathy is the cause of death in 25–30% of diabetics diagnosed before they are 30 years of age.

Almost 90% of diabetics are affected by some degree of retinopathy during the course of their disease. **Proliferative retinopathy**, characterized by the formation of fragile new blood vessels in response to retinal ischaemia, is an asymptomatic but nevertheless ominous development that, if untreated, leads to retinal and vitreous haemorrhage, scar formation and subsequent retinal detachment. Diabetes is the leading cause of blindness in the developed world.

Basic science

Vision

Vision, the reception of light information, the transmission of the evoked response to the visual cortex and the processing and interpretation of the signal, constitutes an immensely complex process.

The eyes are protected by a mucin-containing tear film produced by the lachrymal glands and spread by blinking. Light passes through the pupil, lens and vitreous humour, through the ganglion cell and bipolar cell nerve layers at the front of the retina and is focused on the rod and cone cells in the deeper retinal layer. The pigmented choroid against which the rods and cones rest prevents light reflection onto the photoreceptive cells and image blurring. The rods are more sensitive photoreceptors than cones, but unlike cone cells are unable to resolve detail or determine colour.

Visual acuity is greatest at the macula (the location of the fovea centralis), a thinned area packed with cone cells. The optic nerve leaves the eye at the optic disc which, being devoid of visual receptors, gives rise to the 'blind spot'. Nerve fibres from the macular region lie centrally within the optic nerve. Fibres subserving the upper temporal visual field run in the inferior medial quadrant of the optic nerve. At the optic chiasm, the medial and macular fibres of the optic nerve decussate, and compression of the chiasm from its inferior surface produces bilateral upper temporal field loss which gradually extends downwards to give rise to a complete bitemporal hemianopia (tunnel vision).

After decussation, the visual fibres enter the optic tract and rotate 90° inwards, bringing the fibres subserving the nasal fields to the top of the tract. Unilateral optic tract damage will cause a partial or complete contralateral homonymous hemianopia. The optic tracts enter the lateral geniculate bodies at the top of the brain stem and emerge as the optic radiation, which sweeps around the trigone of the lateral ventricles, inferoposterior to the capsules. Fibres carrying the upper temporal visual field information sweep forward and down into the temporal lobes before running posteriorly to the occipital cortex. Fibres subserving the lower visual fields run more directly backwards into the parietal lobes before reaching the occipital cortex. The visual cortex and much of the optic radiation are supplied largely by the posterior cerebral arteries. The area receiving macular input, however, has a middle cerebral artery supply.

Blindness

The most common causes of sudden visual loss in the developed world are related to vascular events, such as vitreous haemorrhage in proliferative diabetic retinopathy, retinal artery occlusion (transient in amaurosis fugax or permanent in temporal arteritis or polyarteritis nodosa) or retinal vein thrombosis. Retinal detachment, acute optic neuritis, migraine or trauma can also cause sudden visual loss. Rarely, a dense cataract can rapidly condense and acute glaucoma can markedly impair vision. Perhaps the most common cause of blindness worldwide, apart from cataract formation and corneal opacification due to trachoma, is river blindness—infection with *Onchocerca volvulus*. The adult worms, which are 2–3 cm in length, live in painless, mobile, subcutaneous nodules. The microfilariae spread throughout the body under the skin causing a pruritic skin rash, sclerosing lymphadenitis and ocular lesions. One in 20 people with onchocerciasis are blinded by the condition and, in badly affected areas, up to 50% of the population are blinded by the condition before they die.

Causes of retinal haemorrhage

- Diabetes mellitus.
- Hypertension.
- Raised intracranial pressure.
- Retinal vein thrombosis.
- Trauma and retinal detachment.
- Arteritis (polyarteritis nodosa, temporal arteritis).
- Subarachnoid haemorrhage (subhyaloid haemorrhages).
- Subacute bacterial endocarditis.
- Bleeding diathesis.

MCQs

1 Clinically significant proteinuria is often seen within 5 years of diagnosis of diabetes.
2 Proteinuria at 0.5 g per day in diabetics predicts end-stage renal failure or death within 15 years.
3 Temporal arteritis and polyarteritis nodosa are leading causes of blindness worldwide.
4 Diabetic retinopathy is improved in the short term by tightening blood glucose control.
5 The familial risk of insulin-dependent diabetes is greater than that of non-insulin-dependent diabetes.

Case 26
The snoring that stopped

History

A 44-year-old carpenter was referred to the endocrine clinic with a history of pains in both hands that had gradually increased in severity over the previous year. He frequently had to put his hammer down while working, and was beginning to find that even very mild sustained effort, such as holding a newspaper or a steering wheel, caused discomfort. He was also troubled by tiredness and headaches which he attributed to poor sleep and sinusitis, respectively. His wife complained regularly about his loud snoring and, on a few occasions, was even more worried when the noise abruptly stopped. After some time had passed, she would feel obliged to 'give him a little nudge' and the snoring would resume. His only other problem was discomfort in the shoulders which had been put down to the strain of his job.

Physically, he had not noticed any changes except that his feet had 'spread slightly' and that his shoe size had increased accordingly. He was coarse featured on examination, with a slightly bulbous enlargement of the end of the nose and deep frown lines. His hands and feet were broad and the skin was slightly thickened. Crepitus was noted on abduction of his right shoulder. His blood pressure was 174/98 mmHg. Visual fields were full to confrontation.

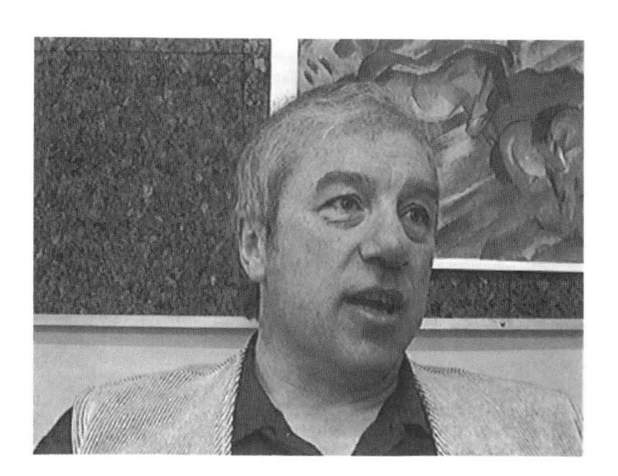

Notes

The patient had acromegaly.

Taken together, the symptoms and signs are very characteristic of acromegaly. Taken individually, however, the symptoms could be attributed to much more common conditions, such as osteoarthritis, obesity, stress or to the process of ageing itself. Once the diagnosis is eventually made, symptoms and signs attributable to acromegaly can typically be traced back over 3 years in the majority of patients.

Acromegaly is caused by the presence of a growth hormone-secreting tumour of the anterior pituitary (somatotrophic adenoma) that develops after puberty. The occurrence of such a tumour before the bony epiphyses have fused (at the end of puberty) gives rise to gigantism, an exceptionally rare condition. Although coarsening of the facial features, headaches, sweating and a progressive increase in jaw, glove, ring and shoe size are well-known features of excess growth hormone, the most common and troublesome symptoms are:

- carpal tunnel syndrome,
- obstructive sleep apnoea, and
- osteoarthritis.

Basic science

Carpal tunnel syndrome

Thickened soft tissues around the **carpal tunnel** compress the median nerve which supplies the two radial lumbricales and the opponens pollicis, flexor pollicis brevis (with the

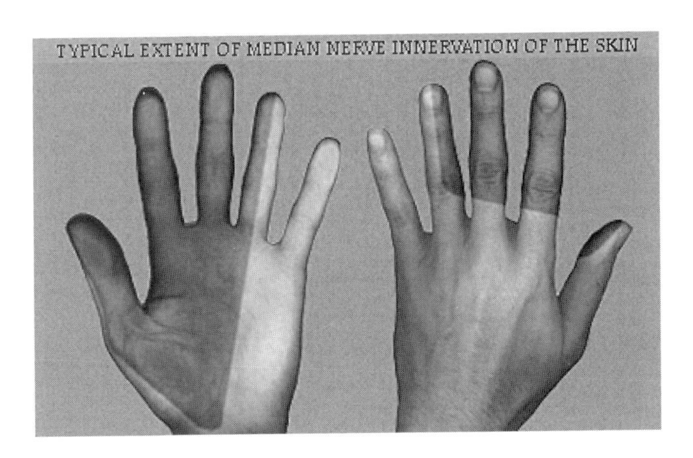

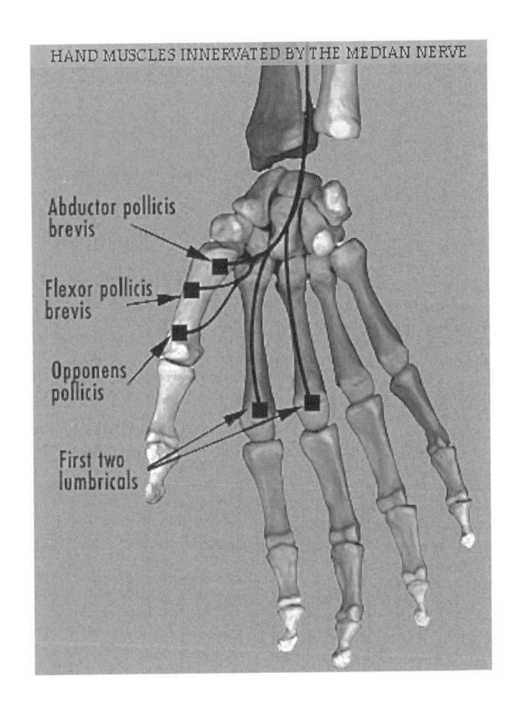

ulnar nerve) and the abductor pollicis brevis. Although the area of sensory loss is confined to the radial side of the palm and the tips of the thumb, index and middle fingers, the pain from carpal tunnel syndrome often extends up the arm and tends to wake the patient at night. The pain can sometimes be reproduced by sustained flexion of the wrist or by tapping the wrist over the median nerve with a tendon hammer. The most common conditions associated with carpal tunnel syndrome are:

- hypothyroidism,
- rheumatoid arthritis,
- pregnancy and the contraceptive pill,
- osteoarthritis of the bones of the wrist, and
- acromegaly.

Obstructive sleep apnoea

Thickening of the tissues of the nasopharynx predisposes to severe snoring and frequent episodes of complete obstruction of the airways during the night. This leads to arterial blood oxygen desaturation and increasing respiratory effort until eventually airflow resumes. Episodes of apnoea are often associated with partial wakefulness, and the patient frequently complains of tiredness in the morning. Obstructive sleep apnoea has also been implicated in the pathogenesis of hypertension, which affects over one-third of acromegalics.

Osteoarthritis

Inappropriate growth of articular cartilage in acromegaly predisposes to osteoarthritis in large joints, such as the hips and knees, and in joints such as the elbows and shoulders that are not usually affected by the disease unless traumatized.

MCQs

1 Carpal tunnel syndrome and obstructive sleep apnoea are typical features of acromegaly.
2 Carpal tunnel syndrome tends to spare the thumb and index finger.
3 Prognathism—forward movement of the lower jaw—is characteristic of acromegaly.
4 Hypertension is a common feature of acromegaly.
5 Visual failure is a typical presenting complaint in acromegaly.

Case 27
The weed that fought back

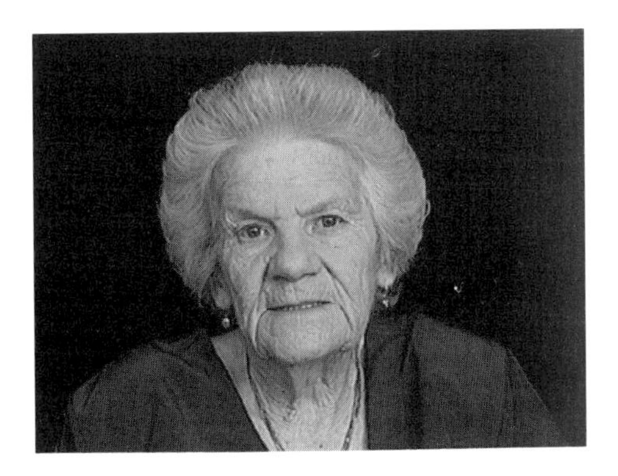

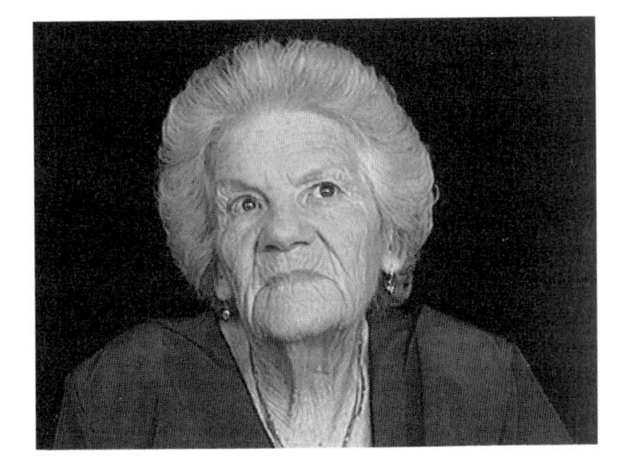

History

A 73-year-old lady was admitted to casualty with a short history of severe pain in the left flank that came on suddenly as she was trying to pull a weed out in the garden. The pain markedly restricted her movement and was worse on deep inspiration. She had previously been completely well and had no previous history of chest pain. She admitted, however, that over the preceding 5 years she had lost almost 3 in in height, but that this had not been associated with any discomfort. Her menopause was at 48 years. On examination, she was found to have an exquisitely tender area overlying a rib and a marked kyphosis. A chest X-ray in casualty demonstrated a spontaneous rib fracture, with no evidence of tumour infiltration locally or elsewhere in the skeleton. A number of vertebrae had wedge fractures and others showed compression deformities. Investigations revealed a normal full blood count, calcium, phosphate and serum proteins, with a marginally elevated alkaline phosphatase level. A formal bone mineral density scan was not carried out. She was treated with rest and analgesics and, over the subsequent 6 weeks, the severe pain gradually diminished to leave her with a dull ache that was exacerbated by activities that required maintaining a standing posture, such as ironing, dressing, washing up, hanging out the washing and making the bed.

Notes

The patient had postmenopausal osteoporosis, and sustained a fractured rib during the relatively trivial task of pulling up a weed.

Osteoporosis affects one in three women and one in 10 men by the age of 70 years. By the age of 80 years, osteoporosis is almost universal in women who did not take sex hormone replacement therapy after the menopause. Even in women who take sex hormone replacement therapy, the risk of fracture returns to untreated control levels within 1 year of cessation of treatment. At the age of 50 years, the lifetime risk of sustaining an osteoporotic fracture is almost 40% for a woman (14% at the hip, 11% at the spine and 13% at the wrist) and 15% for a man.

Osteoporosis is defined as a bone mineral density more than 2.5 standard deviations below the young normal mean (the T score). The T score rather than the Z score (comparison with what would be expected for a person of that age) is usually used as it provides an absolute rather than relative estimate of the risk of fracture. Dual energy X-ray absorptiometry (DEXA) is the most precise method of estimating bone mineral density (±1%).

Basic science

Bone is continuously remodelled by a process of osteoclastic resorption and osteoblastic bone formation at a rate of about 10% per year. An imbalance between bone formation and loss leads to thinning and disruption of the trabecular plates, loss of trabecular continuity and a reduction in bone strength that is disproportionate to the amount of bone lost. The result is an increased risk of fracture, particularly at sites with more than 50% trabecular bone, such as the forearm, hip and vertebrae. Genetics is the most important determining factor of osteoporotic risk. Approximately 85% of the determinant of lumbar bone density is heritable. Biochemical measures of bone resorption are:

- pyridinium cross-links, and
- hydroxyproline,

and measures of formation are:

- alkaline phosphatase (bone isoenzyme), and
- a timed urine collection for osteocalcin.

Calcium homeostasis

Under normal circumstances, circulating total calcium (2.12–2.62 mmol L^{-1}, 9–11 mg/100 mL) and ionized calcium (1.1–1.4 mmol L^{-1}, 4.5–5.6 mg/100 mL) are tightly regulated by the actions of parathyroid hormone and vitamin D (1,25-dihydroxycholecalciferol). A decrease in extracellular calcium ion concentration leads to a very rapid increase in parathyroid hormone secretion from the parathyroid chief cells. Within minutes, this acts on the distal renal tubules to enhance calcium absorption (and increase phosphate loss) and, within an hour or two, stimulates the activity of osteoclasts causing the influx of calcium (and phosphate) into the circulation from the skeleton. A delayed effect of more prolonged parathyroid hormone release is the stimulation of 1α-hydroxylase activity in the proximal tubular cells, which enhances the production of activated vitamin D. Vitamin D stimulates skeletal bone turnover, but has a principal effect of enhancing calcium absorption from the gastrointestinal tract. The increase in circulating calcium levels reduces parathyroid hormone levels to normal by action on parathyroid calcium ion receptors (as distinct from calcium channels). A number of other tissues, such as the kidney, thyroid C cells (which produce calcitonin in response to an increase in calcium), pituitary, brain, lung, testis and ileum, also express calcium ion receptors. Genetic abnormalities of the calcium receptor are responsible for familial benign hypocalciuric hypercalcaemia, autosomal dominant hypocalcaemia with hypercalciuria and neonatal severe hyperparathyroidism. About 10% of patients whose parathyroid glands are explored surgically for presumed primary hyperparathyroidism are found to have familial benign hypocalciuric hypercalcaemia.

Osteomalacia and rickets

Osteomalacia and rickets are caused by a lack of calcium in the diet or, more usually, by a lack of vitamin D or vitamin D effect, because of dietary deficiency, malabsorption or impaired vitamin D action at the bone interface. Osteomalacia in childhood is known as rickets, and is characterized by a restless, irritable baby with hypotonic muscles and abdominal distension. Motor milestones, such as sitting, crawling and standing, occur late, as does eruption of the teeth, and bowing of the legs, predisposition to infections and deformities of the rib cage, pelvis and skull are common. A particularly useful sign of failure of calcification of the osteoid of the developing skull (craniotabes) is a feeling that the skull 'gives' slightly on pressure, like a table tennis ball deforming and springing back. As unfortified human or cows' milk is a poor source of vitamin D, and babies tend to be kept wrapped up and away from sunlight, the condition used to occur particularly in the first year of life. The age group typically affected in affluent countries is 1–3 years, but better nutrition of pregnant and nursing mothers and the fortification of cereals and dairy products, such as margarine and evaporated milk, have made the disease very rare. The typical biochemical picture is:

- low calcium,
- low phosphate, and
- raised alkaline phosphatase levels (a marker of osteoblast activity).

X-ray of the wrist shows characteristic changes at the epiphyses, with blurred outlines of the joint, a widened epiphyseal line and, in older children, the classical concavity of the end of the radius.

In vitamin D-resistant rickets, ordinary therapeutic doses of vitamin D are ineffective in treating the condition. There are a number of causes of the condition, such as a renal tubular defect resulting in phosphate loss, failure to hydroxylate vitamin D in chronic renal failure or malabsorption of vitamin D.

Vitamin D

Vitamin D is a chemically distinct, heat-stable sterol present in fat-containing animal products. The highest natural levels occur in fatty fish and their liver oils. The daily requirement in the diet depends on the amount of skin exposure to sunlight, as vitamin D precursors can be synthesized in the skin in response to sunlight. The daily requirement of vitamin D is around 100 IU (and about four times that in pregnancy and early childhood), and the recommended daily intake is about 400 IU. Cholecalciferol, the dietary form of vitamin D, is inactive until hydroxylated in the liver at the 25 position (25-hydroxycholecalciferol) and further hydroxylated at the 1 position in the kidneys (to 1,25 dihydroxycholecalciferol). Activated vitamin D facilitates calcium absorption from the gut and, in combination with parathyroid hormone, mobilizes calcium from bones.

MCQs

1 A DEXA scan is required to make a diagnosis of osteoporosis.
2 Bone is remodelled at the rate of 50% per year.
3 The most important determinants of osteoporotic risk are menstrual history and age of menopause.
4 Pyridinium cross-links and hydroxyproline are measures of bone resorption.
5 Parathyroid hormone enhances the production of activated vitamin D.

Case 28
Tiredness, palpitations and insomnia

History

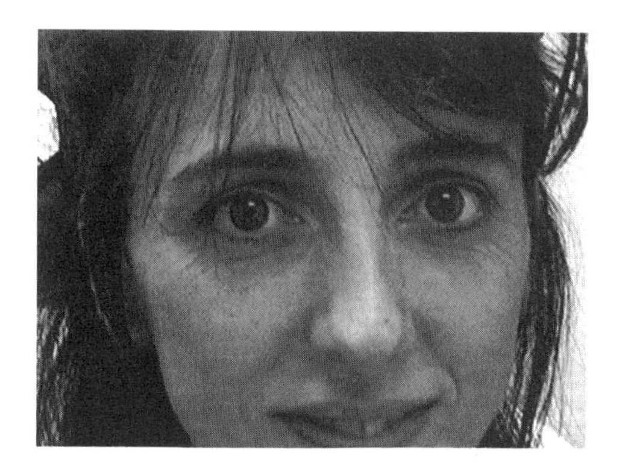

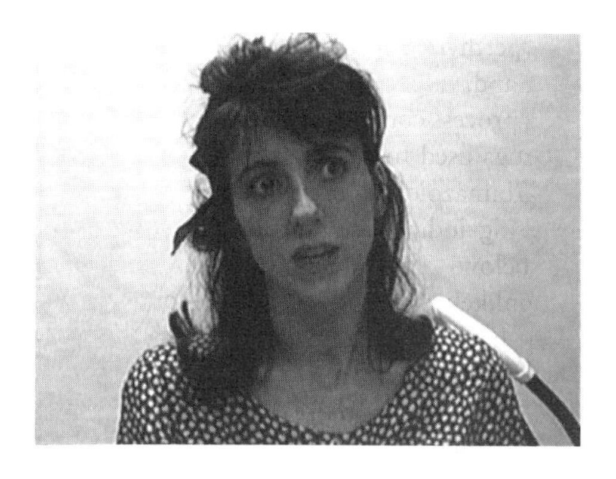

A 23-year-old accounts clerk was seen in clinic with a 6-month history of tiredness, insomnia and palpitations. She complained that her eyes were gritty in the morning, and that her partner and family were finding her mood swings difficult to cope with. Her muscles ached when she ascended stairs and, on undertaking fairly trivial exercise, her heart seemed to race inappropriately. Direct questioning revealed that her weight was steady, but that her menstrual periods had become rather light.

On examination, her blood pressure was 104/78 mmHg with a regular pulse of 92 beats per minute. She was noted to have a fine tremor of the outstretched hands, lid lag and a systolic bruit on auscultation of the thyroid. The thyroid itself was normal in size and smooth and painless on palpation.

Investigations revealed a thyroid-stimulating hormone (TSH) level of <0.1 nmol L^{-1} (normal range = 0.3–6 nmol L^{-1}) and free thyroxine (T4) level of 26.8 nmol L^{-1} (10–23 nmol L^{-1}). Thyroid microsomal antibodies were positive at 1 : 1000.

Notes

The patient had Graves' disease (autoimmune thyrotoxicosis).

Patients with thyrotoxicosis often wear fewer layers of clothing than other patients and tend to be argumentative and short tempered. Retraction of their eyelids exposes the sclera above and sometimes below the cornea and, when following a descending target, downturn of the globe anticipates lowering of the upper eyelid (lid lag). A thyrotoxic proximal myopathy leads to aching of the thighs, particularly on ascending stairs, and, although often tired, patients with thyrotoxicosis may complain of difficulty in sleeping. Frequently, a gradual increase in appetite compensates or overcompensates for increased metabolic demand, and weight changes little until the condition is treated. Loose stools are a relatively infrequent association, and the most classical symptoms of all, finger clubbing (acropachy) and thickening of the pretibial skin (pretibial myxoedema), are rare.

Surgery offers the potential for a rapid and permanent reduction in thyroid hormone levels to normal. Specific disadvantages added to the usual complications of surgery and

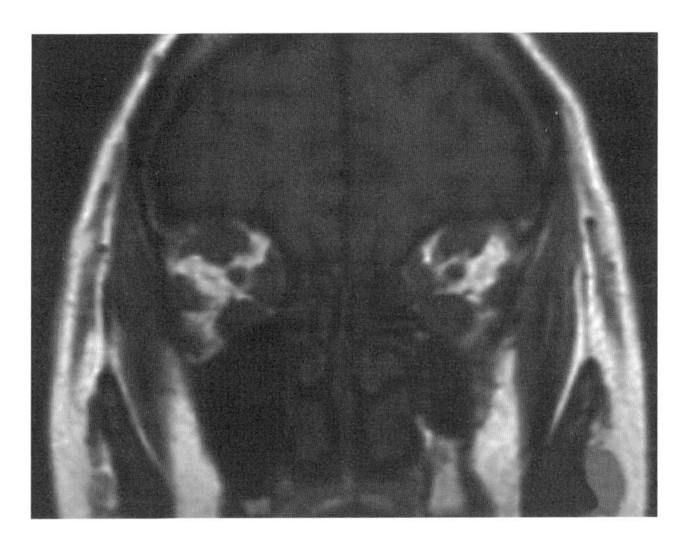

anaesthesia are damage to the recurrent laryngeal nerves or parathyroid glands, and the development of hypothyroidism or recurrence of hyperthyroidism if too much or too little of the gland, respectively, is resected. The underlying process continues unabated.

Drugs used to control thyrotoxicosis, such as carbimazole and propylthiouracil, work by blocking iodine trapping and organification (see below). They are almost always effective, but unlikely to alter the course of the disease. They have to be taken in the longer term and can produce idiosyncratic side-effects, such as rash or, more seriously, profound neutropenia.

Radioiodine permanently reduces the activity of the thyroid gland. It is an extremely low risk but relatively slow acting antithyroid treatment that is not associated with an increase in the risk of inducing thyroid malignancy. The dose is idiosyncratic and difficult to judge. Many patients end up hypothyroid and require long-term thyroid hormone replacement therapy.

Basic science

Formation of thyroid hormones

Iodine is present in seafood, iodized salt, meat and vegetables. The amount in animal foods depends on the level in the animals' diets, and the amount in vegetables and cereals on the soil levels of iodine. Iodine is actively transported into the thyroid gland (trapped) and rapidly oxidized by thyroid peroxidase to form a series of iodinated proteins (organification), principally thyroglobulin, in a reaction that is stimulated by TSH and inhibited by many antithyroid drugs. Thyroglobulin, the principal component of the colloid within thyroid follicles, is hydrolysed by proteases and cleaved by peptidases to yield mono- and diiodotyrosine. These are coupled together to form the active thyroid hormones triiodothyronine (T3) and tetraiodothyronine (thyroxine or T4) that are released into the circulation. In blood, T4 and T3 are almost entirely bound to thyroid-binding globulin, thyroid-binding prealbumin and albumin. The remaining 'free' hormone is available to act on the tissues at the nuclear and mitochondrial level via thyroid hormone receptors to influence growth, differentiation and energy expenditure.

MCQs

1 In the thyroid, trapped iodine is oxidized by peroxidase to form thyroglobulin.
2 Triiodothyronine is produced in the

thyroid principally by deiodination of thyroxine.

3 Common symptoms of thyrotoxicosis include pretibial myxoedema and acropachy.

4 Lid lag is failure to fully elevate the upper lid on upward gaze.

5 Lid retraction is a specific sign of autoimmune thyrotoxicosis (Graves' disease).

Case 29
Vomiting and abdominal pain

History

A 38-year-old production designer was admitted to hospital with a 20-h history of nausea, vomiting and abdominal discomfort. She denied any dietary indiscretions, had not felt unwell in the recent past and had not been in contact with anyone who was experiencing or had subsequently experienced similar symptoms. Insulin-dependent diabetes mellitus had been diagnosed at the age of 18 years, when she presented with a history of thirst and weight loss, and, after a honeymoon period lasting 4 months, during which she stuck rigorously to a macrobiotic diet and lost even more weight, she was stabilized on insulin and subsequently remained completely well on four injections of insulin daily. Her blood glucose levels varied between 4 and 7 mmol L^{-1} (normal range = 3–7 mmol L^{-1}) and, despite this exemplary level of control, she had only once become symptomatically hypoglycaemic. She had continued to inject herself with her usual dose of insulin throughout the very recent episode of abdominal pain and uncontrollable vomiting, and was very surprised to find that her blood glucose had risen to 28 mmol L^{-1} prior to admission to hospital.

The elevated blood glucose was confirmed on admission, and was found to be associated with marked ketonuria and acidosis, with a blood pH of 7.2 and levels of HCO_3^- of 13 mmol L^{-1}, Na^+ of 145 mmol L^{-1} and K^+ of 4 mmol L^{-1}. There was no evidence of diabetic nephropathy, neuropathy or retinopathy on examination. She was treated with intravenous saline and insulin with potassium replacement when appropriate, and made a rapid, uneventful recovery.

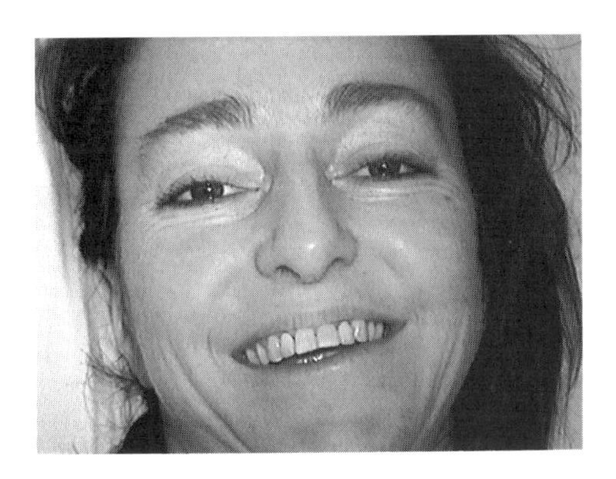

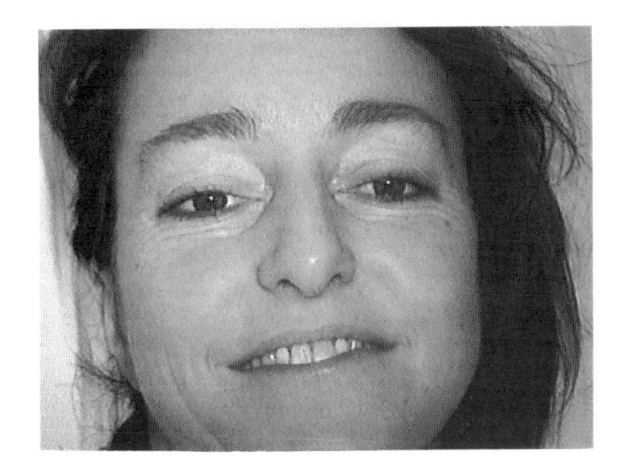

Notes

The patient had developed diabetic ketoacidosis.

The acidosis of ketone body accumulation, together with dehydration caused by nausea, vomiting and continued polyuria, leads to:

- tachycardia and hypotension with peripheral vasodilatation,
- decreased core temperature and a warm periphery,
- thirst,
- nocturia,
- polydipsia,

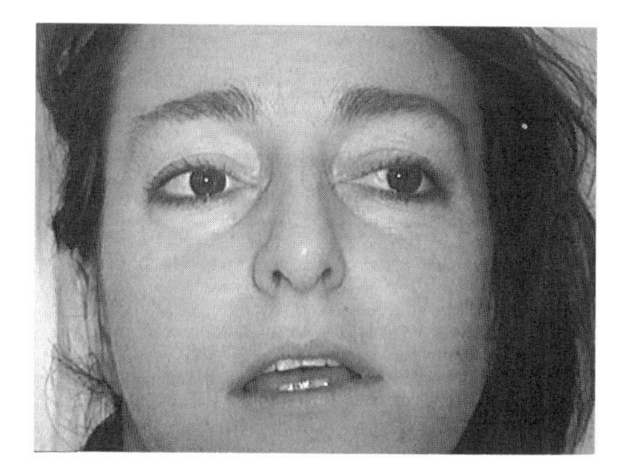

- abdominal pain,
- the finding of ketones in the urine and a metabolic acidosis (arterial blood pH <7.25 and bicarbonate <15 mmol L^{-1}) with elevated glucose (characteristically >16 mmol L^{-1} (>290 mg/100 mL)) confirm the diagnosis.

Lack of insulin leads to a rapid rise in hepatic glucose output and a fall in peripheral glucose uptake. In the absence of insulin, free fatty acids from adipose stores and hepatic fatty acid oxidation lead to high circulating levels of acetoacetic and β-hydroxybutyric acids.

Basic science

Fuel metabolism

In simple terms, oxidation of energy-containing ingested foodstuffs to carbon dioxide and water is accompanied by adenosine triphosphate (ATP) generation, which is used as the principal high energy substrate of the body.

When calorific intake exceeds immediate demand, excess energy-containing substrate is stored as fat, glycogen and structural protein. Between meals, when energy demand exceeds calorific intake, these substrates are mobilized through the smooth, integrated transition between anabolic and catabolic metabolic states. In essence, a high insulin to glucagon ratio is chiefly responsible for the anabolic state, while a low insulin to glucagon ratio initiates catabolism.

Following the ingestion of carbohydrates, intraluminal and brush border enzymes in the intestines break them down to their constituent sugars, which are absorbed and reach the liver via the portal vein. More than 60% of the glucose is immediately utilized for glycogen synthesis by the liver, the remainder entering the systemic circulation as glucose, with small amounts of the glucose oxidation products, lactate and pyruvate. As blood glucose concentrations rise, insulin release from the pancreas increases and glucagon concentrations fall, accelerating hepatic glycogen formation and increasing the disposal of glucose in muscle (as glycogen and substrate for direct oxidation) and in adipose tissue (as a substrate for long chain fatty acid synthesis and esterification with glucose-derived glycerol to form triglycerides). Triglycerides are also formed by the liver and transported to adipose tissue in the form of very low density lipoproteins.

Glycolysis is the oxidative breakdown reaction sequence that carries glucose to pyruvate through glucose-6-phosphate, fructose-6-phosphate, fructose-1,6-diphosphate, 3-phosphoglyceraldehyde, 1,3-diphosphoglycerate, 3-phosphoglycerate and phosphoenolpyruvate. Pyruvate is then converted by thiamine to acetyl-coenzyme A, which is a central biochemical starting material for fatty acid synthesis and is the fuel for the citric acid cycle (Krebs' cycle), the chief metabolic furnace of the body. In one turn of the cycle, a pair of carbon atoms, fed in as acetate (acetyl-coenzyme A), combines with four-carbon oxaloacetic acid to form six-carbon citrate, from which two molecules of carbon dioxide are released. Four pairs of hydrogen atoms are released and channelled into auxiliary reactions that overall produce 12 molecules of ATP from adenosine diphosphate (ADP) per molecule of acetyl-coenzyme A completely oxidized.

Vomiting

Nausea and vomiting are common, important and distressing symptoms. They are frequently caused by the metabolic consequences of ketoacidosis.

Nausea, the feeling of the desire to vomit, is usually accompanied by anorexia and changes in autonomic activity that lead to reduced gastric activity, altered duodenal and small intestinal motility, skin pallor, sweating, increased salivation and, sometimes, bradycardia and hypotension. Vomiting, the forceful expulsion of gastric contents through the mouth, is largely brought about by contraction of the diaphragm and abdominal musculature with relaxation of the gastric fundus, rather than through an active gastric process. Forceful vomiting (projectile vomiting) suggests complete gastric outflow obstruction in babies or raised intracranial pressure in adults, and repeated vomiting, particularly if forceful/vigorous, can rupture the oesophagus or cause linear mucosal tears at the junction of the oesophagus and stomach, leading to haematemesis (Mallory–Weiss syndrome). Repeated vomiting leads to dehydration, metabolic alkalosis and hypokalaemia, and the acidity of gastric contents can damage dentition and predispose to aspiration of gastric contents with pneumonitis.

The process of vomiting is under the control of neural centres in the brain stem medulla close to visceral autonomic centres. Dopamine receptors in the medulla activate the chemotactic trigger zone, and dopamine antagonists, such as phenothiazine derivatives (e.g. metoclopramide and prochlorperazine), inhibit it. In addition, specific ($5HT_3$) serotonin antagonists (such as Ondansetron and Granisetron) also art centrally to control nausea and vomiting.

MCQs

1 An increase in circulating insulin leads to a rapid rise in hepatic glucose output.
2 The presence of ketones in the urine is diagnostic of diabetic ketoacidosis.
3 Diabetic ketoacidosis can be reversed without insulin.
4 Vomiting is caused by powerful contractions of the stomach.
5 Vomiting damages dentition.

Case 30
Weakness, weight loss and polyuria

History

A 33-year-old lead singer in a band was seen in the outpatient department with a 5-week history of feeling generally unwell and a 1-week history of thirst, polyuria, nocturia and occasional episodes of dysuria. In retrospect, the history may have extended back more than 1 year, during which time, despite eating normally, he gradually lost weight and seemed to have less energy than before. To some extent these changes were put down to his frenetic and unhealthy life on the road, even though the patient had always made an effort to look after himself. Several months before his presentation, the patient had an attack of influenza and seemed to suffer symptoms out of proportion to the severity of the illness. He had also noticed once or twice that his vision seemed blurred and that his colour vision had changed, although like his other symptoms these observations were difficult to put into context at the time.

This patient did not want his face to appear

Notes

The patient had developed insulin-dependent diabetes mellitus.

The gradual destruction of pancreatic β cells, that led inexorably to absolute insulin deficiency, started many months before his initial symptoms of weight loss and reduced energy. His predisposition to infections may have resulted from this, and variable hyperglycaemia changed the osmotic tension in his aqueous and vitreous humour, leading to refractive changes and transient blurred vision. The transient changes in colour vision that the patient observed are more difficult to put into context. After a fast lasting ≥8 h, a blood glucose level of >7.0 mmol L^{-1} (>127 mg/100 mL) is diagnostic of diabetes, and is now thought to be a more specific and reproducible diagnostic test than either a full glucose tolerance test or a single blood glucose estimation 2 h after a 75-g oral glucose load.

Basic science

Islet cell function

The adult pancreas contains around 2 000 000 islets, each of which consists of a mixed population of several hundred thousand cells secreting glucagon (α cells), insulin (β cells), somatostatin (δ cells) or pancreatic polypeptide. Approximately 80% of the cells are insulin producing, and there is good evidence of the important paracrine effects of this peptide on the secretory activity of adjacent cells. Insulin secretion is increased by an increase in blood glucose, and is also modified by parasympathetic and sympathetic innervation and by levels of acetylcholine, noradrenaline, adrenaline and other neuropeptides, such as galanin and vasoactive intestinal polypeptide. Sympathetic activity suppresses insulin release and increases glucagon release during exercise, and parasympathetic activity may be involved in the stimulation of insulin release associated with food ingestion. Pancreatic polypeptide, which modifies gastrointestinal motility, is released principally through vagal nerve activity. Somatostatin, which is also produced in many sites throughout the central nervous system, inhibits endocrine and exocrine pancreatic secretion.

MCQs

1 The pathological and biochemical abnormalities of insulin-dependent diabetes start simultaneously.
2 Sympathetic stimulation suppresses insulin secretion.
3 An abnormal glucose tolerance test is a prerequisite for the diagnosis of diabetes mellitus.
4 Insulin secreted from β cells can influence the secretory activity of other islet cells.
5 Approximately 50% of islet cells are insulin-secreting β cells.

Case 31
An unexpected fall on the way out of bed

History

A 67-year-old retired artist was admitted with a history of sudden onset of weakness in his legs. He had been well until the previous week, when he developed influenza-like symptoms. On the sixth day after the start of symptoms, he noticed that he had to struggle a little to reach the top of the stairs, but he put this down to the 'weakness, aches and pains' that would be expected with a virus infection. In the early hours of the following morning, he attempted to get out of bed to pass water. To his surprise, he fell to the ground without managing to stand, and found himself unable to get back into bed. His wife helped him into bed and called for an ambulance.

In accident and emergency the patient looked well and was able to give a full history. On examination, he had bilateral, flaccid paraparesis (weakness of both legs) with reduced ankle jerks and normal sensation. When reviewed the following day, his arms, which had been unaffected on presentation, were also found to have markedly reduced muscle power and hyporeflexia.

A lumbar puncture revealed a marked increase in protein with no increase in cells.

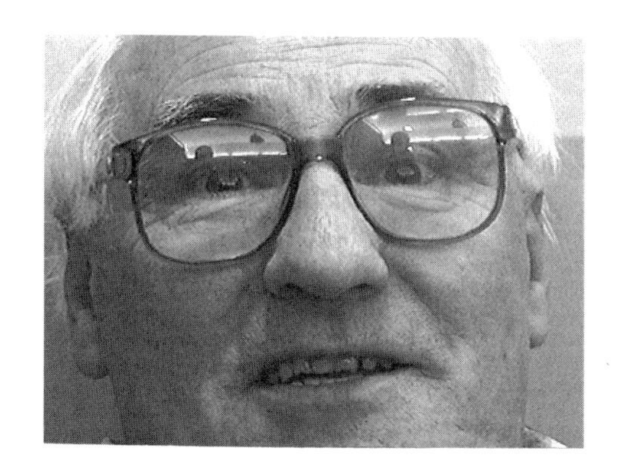

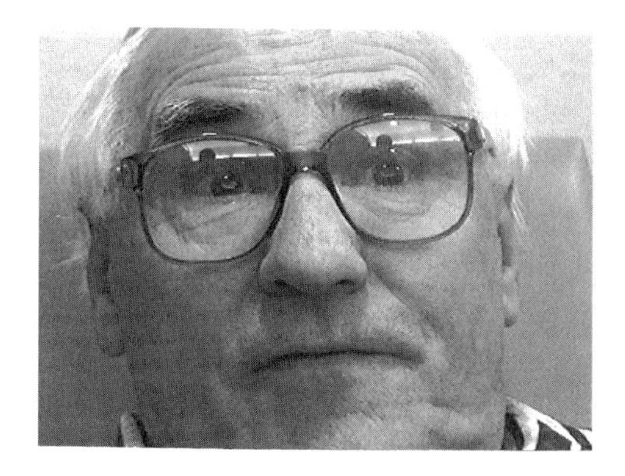

Notes

The patient had developed Guillain–Barré syndrome.

After a brief spell on the receiving ward, he was transferred to intensive care where the weakness progressively worsened for 2 days. He denied any respiratory and speech problems at any time. Over a period of a year, he made an almost complete recovery that started with the return of strength to his hands and later his feet.

Guillain–Barré syndrome is an acute, immune-mediated, demyelinating polyneuropathy. Its annual incidence of between 1 and 2 per 100 000 makes it the most common cause of acute neuromuscular paralysis in the UK. It is usually diagnosed on the basis of the development of symmetrical weakness and loss of tendon reflexes associated, in two-thirds of cases, with an infection. In these cases, the condition usually develops within 2 weeks and always within 4 weeks of the precipitant. Clinical expression varies markedly, with ophthalmoplegia, respiratory and bulbar muscles being involved in some patients. Molecular mimicry is currently thought to be the likely mechanism that triggers off the syndrome. Antibodies against epitopes of *Campylobacter jejuni* strains have been observed in the classical ascending form of the disease, but cytomegalovirus and Epstein–Barr virus account for most of the cases triggered by viruses.

Weakness in two or all four limbs develops over one to several days, and is associated with diminished or absent tendon reflexes and sensory symptoms. The differential diagnosis includes:

- poliomyelitis,
- cauda equina lesions,
- botulism,
- muscle diseases,
- causes of vasculitis, such as systemic lupus erythematosus,
- porphyria,
- diphtheria,
- Lyme disease,
- hypokalaemia, and
- poisoning with alcohol, drugs, heavy metals or organophosphate.

Plasma exchange and high dose immunoglobulins (±methylprednisolone) have been shown to be useful treatment adjuncts to supportive therapy. Approximately 80% of patients make a complete or nearly complete recovery. A further 25% need respiratory support during the illness, 10% are still severely disabled a year after the onset of the condition and, despite treatment, 4–8% of patients die, usually from pulmonary embolism, respiratory failure or cardiac dysrhythmias. Plasma exchange and intravenous immunoglobulin have both been shown to hasten recovery from the condition.

Although axons in the central nervous system have a very limited capacity to regenerate, peripheral nerve regeneration can take place very effectively over a period of months to a year. Peripheral nerve remyelination after a demyelinating injury can occur even more quickly.

Basic science

Myelin

Nerve cell axons are surrounded by Schwann cells, interrupted at millimetre intervals by constrictions known as nodes of Ranvier. Myelinated nerves are characterized by having Schwann cell membranes extensively coiled around the axon to form a thick myelin sheath. Effective electrical insulation by the myelin sheath induces depolarizing conduction to jump between nodes of Ranvier. This so-called saltatory conduction accelerates current flow to 50 times that found in the fastest unmyelinated nerves, which are surrounded by a single layer of Schwann cell plasma membrane only.

Demyelination

Multiple sclerosis and a number of less common conditions, such as acute disseminated and acute necrotizing encephalomyelitis, cause focal inflammation and destruction of myelin sheaths in the central nervous system. Although the exact cause of demyelination is unknown, viral infections and autoimmunity are heavily implicated.

Structure of the motor unit and muscle types

The terminal branching of motor neurone axons ensures that, under normal conditions, they synapse directly with the hundreds of striated muscle cells that constitute a motor unit. Muscles capable of very accurate movement, such as the extraocular muscles, have fewer muscle fibres in each motor unit. For all movements, the strength of contraction increases as more motor units of increasing size are recruited. When motor neurones malfunction, they may depolarize in isolation from surrounding neurones and give rise to fasciculation (visible twitching of muscle) as well as muscular atrophy. Spontaneous contraction of single denervated muscle fibres leads to fibrillation, which can be recorded electromyographically, but cannot be seen through the skin.

There are three types of skeletal (striated) muscle, differing in their energy metabolism, speed of contraction and resistance to fatigue. The two extremes are postural muscles, adapted for continuous, slow, fatigue-resistant contractile activity, and fast-twitch glycolytic muscles, that respond rapidly and powerfully but are quickly fatigued. Postural muscles are small in diameter and red owing to their myoglobin content. Their small diameter and myoglobin content facilitate transfer of oxygen from dense capillary networks to muscle mitochondria. In contrast, fast-twitch (white) glycolytic muscles consist mostly of anaerobic fast fibres that do not contain myoglobin and have few capillaries and mitochondria. Adenosine triphosphate (ATP) can be produced quickly but, once glycogen stores are exhausted, they are rapidly fatigued. The third type of fibre is intermediate between the above two.

MCQs

1 Guillain–Barré syndrome is primarily a virally induced axonal degeneration.
2 Guillain–Barré syndrome may develop as much as 6 weeks after the causative infection.
3 The respiratory muscles are rarely involved in Guillain–Barré syndrome.
4 All but 5% of patients make a complete recovery from Guillain–Barré syndrome.
5 Fast-twitch glycolytic muscles are capable of rapid generation of force.

Case 32
Recurrent facial pain

History

A 57-year-old housewife was seen in clinic with facial pain that started after a troublesome tooth extraction from the right upper jaw. In the same region, she subsequently developed sudden and extremely severe lancinating pains that made her wince or made her whole body 'jump'. The pains would come in flashes and were knife-like in character. Although, at times, facial movement, washing, chewing, drying her face and even speaking seemed to be associated with the onset of pain, this was not usually the case and, under most circumstances, the pain would appear quite abruptly at any time during the day but never at night. The patient rated the pain as more intense and less agreeable than the pain of childbirth.

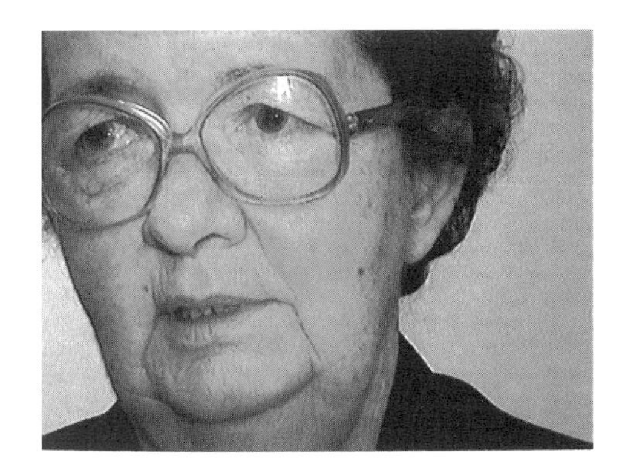

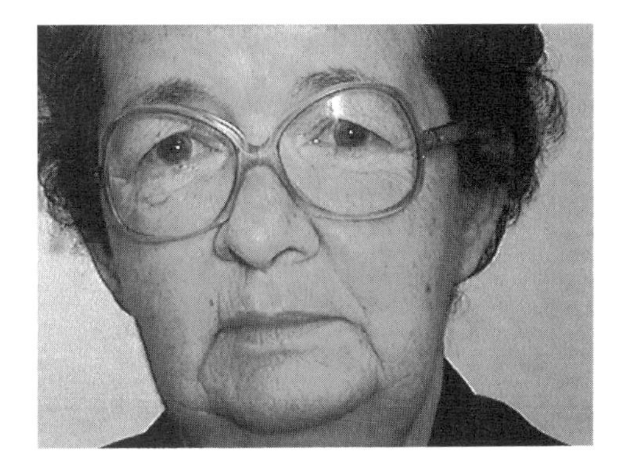

Notes

The patient had trigeminal neuralgia. Carbamazepine treatment markedly reduced the intensity of pain, but did not relieve it completely. Eventually, surgery was carried out to cut branches of the maxillary division of the trigeminal nerve on the right side, since when the pain has been less severe, but not completely controlled.

Trigeminal pain is characteristically lancinating with brief, excruciating paroxysms sometimes occurring in such rapid succession that the patient complains of more prolonged pain. Involvement of the ophthalmic division of the trigeminal nerve, particularly in isolation, is rare. Most cases affect either the maxillary or mandibular division, almost always unilaterally. Characteristically, sensory loss cannot be demonstrated. In many patients, the pain can be triggered by local contact or movement (such as smiling, talking, washing

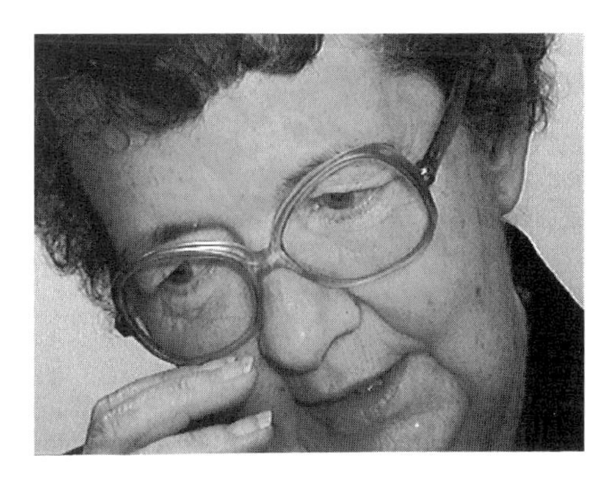

or exposure to the wind), and the whole episode tends to resolve after a few weeks, but the pain recurs subsequently. Glossopharyngeal neuralgia is similar, but manifests through the cutaneous distribution of the glossopharyngeal nerve with pain at the back of the mouth and ear, sometimes triggered by coughing or swallowing.

Basic science

Trigeminal nerve

The trigeminal nerve is the principal sensory nerve for the head and the motor nerve for the muscles of mastication. The extent of sensory innervation is highly significant clinically, as facial numbness is a common symptom in patients with functional rather than organic disease. The important distinguishing features are as follows:

1 The ophthalmic division of the trigeminal nerve extends to the vertex (uppermost part of the head) or just beyond, rather than, as might be assumed, the hairline.

2 As all axial sensory nerves interdigitate in the midline, in unilateral sensory nerve palsy, the line of sensory loss should be a few millimetres from the midline, towards the affected side.

3 The corneal reflex, tested by touching the cornea (not the sclera or eyelashes) to one side of the pupil (so that sight of an object does not induce a blink) with a wisp of cotton wool, is difficult to resist and is an excellent sign of intact innervation.

4 The region of skin over the angle of the jaw is innervated by branches from C2 and C3, not the mandibular division of the trigeminal nerve. Thus, in trigeminal palsy, the sensation over this area should be preserved.

The motor component of the trigeminal nerve, in addition to the muscles of mastication, includes the tensor tympani, tensor veli palatini, anterior belly of digastric and mylohyoid muscles. The significant bilateral innervation to the motor nuclei of the trigeminal nerve tends to make the assessment of motor function less informative than that of sensory function.

Causes of facial pain

Pain referred from the eye. Refractive problems can cause frontal headaches. Optic neuritis may cause pain on moving the eye. Glaucoma tends to cause pain in and around the eye. Scleritis and episcleritis typically cause pain in the eye that radiates back into the side of the head.

Pain referred from the paranasal sinuses. Tenderness of the frontal or maxillary sinuses is common and can sometimes be elicited by local pressure. In ethmoid or sphenoid sinusitis, the pain is more localized behind the nose and is often accompanied by a blocked nose.

Dental pain. Impacted or carious teeth and root abscesses can cause pain in the maxilla or mandible that can radiate into the head.

Ear and temporomandibular joint pain. Pain around the ear suggests either ear infections or temporomandibular joint pain. The latter can sometimes be elicited by jaw movement or biting.

Herpetic neuralgia. Particularly the first division of the trigeminal nerve is a common site for herpes zoster infection. The pain occasionally precedes the skin lesion (if the rash occurs at all) and, unfortunately, may continue as a neuralgic pain after the skin lesions have resolved.

Atypical facial pain. This typically occurs in young women with previous psychiatric morbidity. It is typified by continuous (rather than lancinating) pain in one cheek.

MCQs

1 Involvement of the first division of the trigeminal nerve in neuralgia is typical.
2 Touch sensation over the affected area is temporarily reduced after an attack of neuralgia.
3 The tendency to attacks of trigeminal neuralgia waxes and wanes with time.
4 Atypical facial pain is usually continuous rather than lancinating.
5 Pain radiating into the temporal region is typical of episcleritis.

Case 33
Recurrent 'funny turns'

History

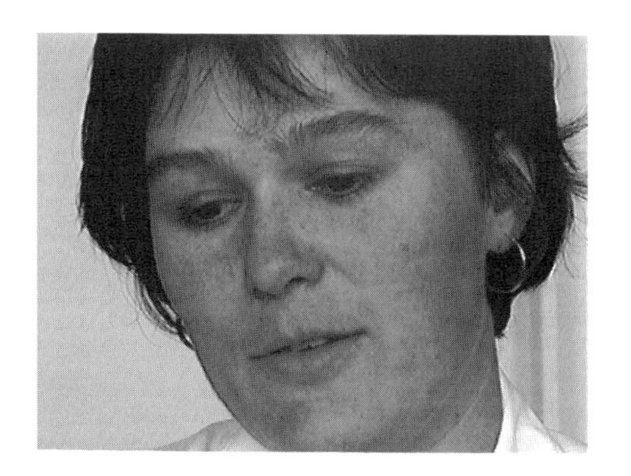

A 25-year-old secretary was seen in clinic with a 3-month history of 'funny turns'. She had previously been entirely well and had no family history of such events. Almost all of the episodes occurred within a few minutes of getting out of bed in the morning, and started as 'a tight feeling of butterflies in the stomach' which would ascend to the chest over a period of a few seconds. Her vision would then 'close in' or be lost completely, and the patient would tend to fall forward without either losing consciousness completely or sustaining an injury. After a minute or two, the whole episode would pass off and she would return completely to normal without any subsequent drowsiness or headache. At no time, according to the patient (and her family), did she lose conscious contact with the environment. As a child, she recalled suffering from *petit mal* epilepsy, diagnosed symptomatically and electroencephalographically, but remembers that she had been told that, on several occasions, she had lost consciousness completely. Treatment with ethosuximide controlled the fits successfully from early childhood until the age of 11 years when, after years of being fit free, the treatment was stopped. The 'funny turns' did not resume until 3 months before her presentation.

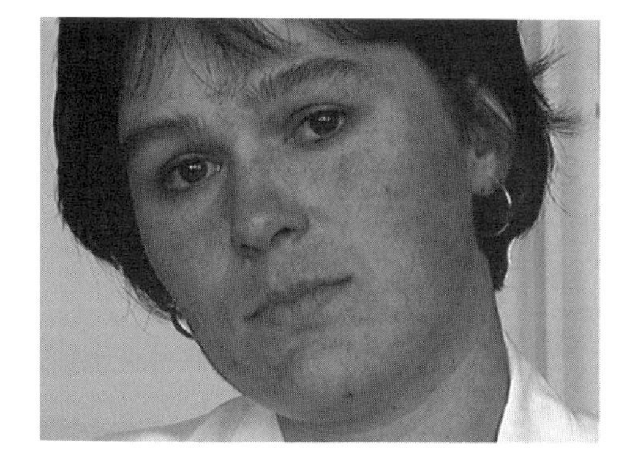

Examination was entirely normal.

Notes

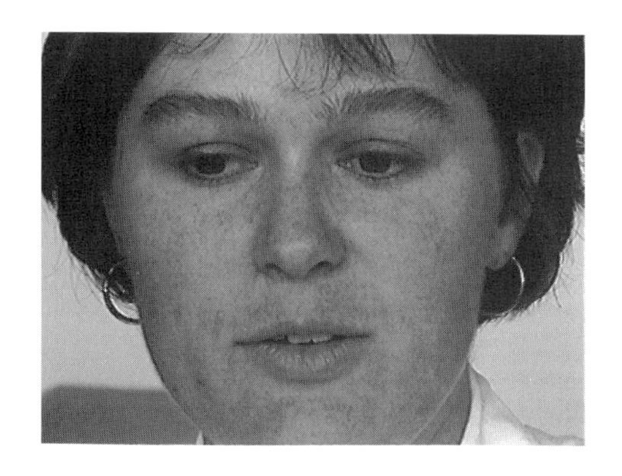

The patient had developed idiopathic simple partial seizures.

Epilepsy refers to a group of neurological conditions characterized by recurrent paroxysmal changes in neurological function caused by abnormal electrical activity. Consciousness and motor function are frequently affected, but emotional, sensory and cognitive changes may also occur. It occurs at any age and affects 0.5–2% of the population. Between seizures, 20% of patients with *petit mal* epilepsy and 40% with *grand mal* epilepsy have normal EEGs, and many that do have EEG abnormalities have non-specific changes only.

In simple partial seizures, motor, sensory, autonomic or psychic signs occur without loss of consciousness or loss of conscious contact with the environment. Typical examples are recurrent contractions of the muscles of one part of the body, paraesthesia, vertigo, auditory or visual hallucinations, *déjà vu* (the feeling of having previously visited a place that is, in fact, quite new) or *jamais vu* (the feeling of visiting a place that seems quite new, but should be very familiar to the patient).

In the episodic behavioural changes that constitute complex partial seizures, the individual loses conscious contact with the environment. Auras, such as unusual smell, *déjà vu*, intense emotion and sensory illusions, such as macropsia (small objects appearing large) or micropsia (the opposite), also occur. In these seizures, the patient's current activity is replaced with minor motor activity such as lip smacking, swallowing, walking aimlessly or even driving a car or playing a musical instrument. After the event, there is often a period of amnesia lasting for several hours before complete recovery.

Both simple and complex partial seizures can generalize with loss of consciousness and convulsive motor activity immediately or after a minute or two. They may not always follow the same pattern, and generalized convulsions with no aura may be interspersed with partial seizures. The presence of an aura or focal feature before the onset of a convulsion is an important pointer towards a focal rather than primary generalized seizure.

Primary generalized seizures

Primary generalized seizures are the most common type of seizure, usually starting without warning with a sudden loss of consciousness. Tonic muscular contraction, including the respiratory muscles, results in incontinence and a cry as air is forced through the closed glottis. The individual falls to the floor in an opisthotonic posture (lordosis and extended neck and limbs), and remains rigid and in a state of respiratory arrest which may lead to cyanosis. After many seconds, the tonic rigidity gives way to a series of clonic rhythmic contractions of all four limbs, which ends after a variable period in complete relaxation, followed by a period of non-rousability lasting minutes or longer. Consciousness accompanied initially by disorientation then gradually returns, with amnesia for the event and sometimes the events leading up to the seizure. Headaches and drowsiness are very common postictal phenomena, and the patient may not return to complete normality for hours or days. In Jacksonian epilepsy, the chaotic electrical activity starts in one part of the motor cortex and propagates along it before generalizing. Afterwards, Todd's palsy, paralysis of the affected limb, can last for up to 3 days.

Febrile convulsions, short, tonic–clonic convulsions, occur in 2–5% of the population of 3 months to 5 years of age. Although harmless in themselves, they must be distinguished from convulsions due to central nervous system infections, such as meningitis or encephalitis.

Absence seizures

Absence seizures consist of the sudden cessation of conscious activity without convulsive activity or loss of postural control, lasting a second or two to minutes, followed by complete recovery without postictal confusion or headaches. There may be minor motor phenomena, such as eyelid fluttering, chewing movements or hand movements, and automatisms during longer fits that mimic complex partial seizures. They begin in childhood and may continue into adulthood. They may occur hundreds of times a day and go on for months before the problem is recognized.

The EEG shows pathognomonic 3-Hz spike and wave discharges synchronously throughout all the leads. One-third of patients outgrow them, one-third continue to have simple absence seizures and one-third go on to occasional concomitant generalized tonic–clonic seizures.

In atypical absence seizures, absence seizures coexist with other forms of generalized seizures, such as tonic, myoclonic or atonic.

Myoclonic seizures

Myoclonic seizures are sudden, brief, single or sometimes repetitive muscle contractions involving one part of the body or the whole body, often accompanied by a fall, but not by loss of consciousness. Myoclonic seizures are usually idiopathic, but may accompany uraemia, hepatic failure, Creutzfeldt–Jakob disease and the leucoencephalopathies.

Atonic seizures

Atonic seizures are brief losses of muscle tone and consciousness without any accompanying tonic activity. They may accompany other types of epilepsy or occur alone.

Other types

Infantile spasms occur up to 1 year of age and consist of brief, synchronous flexion of the neck, torso and arms, often in infants with underlying neurological disease.

Status epilepticus involves prolonged or repetitive seizures, usually tonic–clonic (*grand mal*), without periods of recovery in between. Epilepsy partialis continua is similar, although it affects a body part or region and leaves consciousness intact.

Catamenial epilepsy involves seizures related to the menstrual phase.

Photoconvulsive epilepsy involves seizures related to photic stimulation.

Basic science

Pathophysiology of epilepsy

Although many types of metabolic and anatomic lesions can cause epilepsy, there is at present no known pathognomonic lesion of the epileptic brain. Rhythmic, repetitive, synchronous discharges are seen on EEG, a test that detects composite cortical electrical activity, but is not able to detect electrical events that occur deeper down. A synchronous discharge produces a spike. If it spreads throughout the brain, it produces a generalized seizure.

International classification of epileptic seizures

1 Partial or focal seizures.
   Simple partial seizures (with motor, sensory, autonomic or psychic signs).
   Complex partial seizures (psychomotor or temporal lobe seizures).
   Secondary generalized partial seizures.
2 Primary generalized seizures.
   Tonic–clonic (*grand mal*).
   Tonic.
   Absence (*petit mal*).
   Atypical absence.
   Myoclonic.
   Atonic.
   Infantile spasm.
3 Status epilepticus.
   Tonic–clonic status.
   Absence status.
   Epilepsy partialis continua.
4 Recurrent patterns.
   Sporadic.
   Cyclic.
   Reflex (photomyoclonic, somatosensory, musicogenic, reading epilepsy).

MCQs

1 Simple partial seizures can generalize and lead to loss of consciousness.

2 An aura typically precedes primary generalized seizures (*grand mal* epilepsy).
3 *Petit mal* epilepsy is associated with a focal 3-Hz spike and wave activity on the EEG.
4 One-third of patients with *petit mal* epilepsy in childhood outgrow it.
5 Seizures within the first 24 h of injury are not associated with a poor prognosis.

Case 34
The man with the blunt razor

History

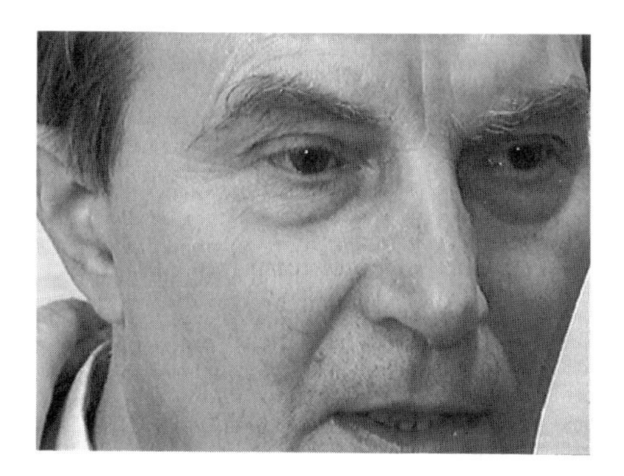

A 67-year-old man was seen in surgery with a history of tremor and depressed mood. He had been well until the age of 58 years, when he noticed that his razor seemed to 'get stuck on his face' while he was trying to shave. This phenomenon gradually increased in frequency. Some months later, he noticed a difficulty in turning over in bed, and had to get out of bed and back in to change sides. His wife first noticed the tremor of his hands and reported that her husband had suffered a series of episodes during which his difficulty initiating movement had dramatically worsened. For the 20–60 min duration of these attacks, he found himself literally stuck to the spot and unable to speak.

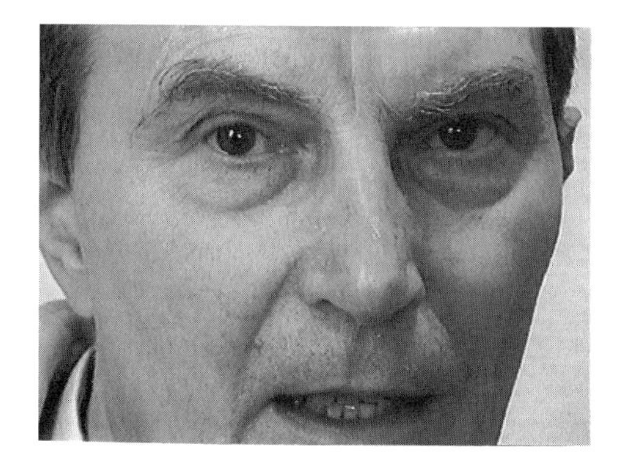

On examination, the patient looked well, but his face was mask-like and devoid of the fine, expressive facial muscle movements that characterize normal basal ganglia function. A slow, rest tremor of his hands, worse on the left, was noted, and his gait, once he got going, was shuffling and tended to accelerate. Moderate 'cogwheel' muscular rigidity was present on examination of his arms and legs. Muscle power was normal, as was his intellectual function.

Notes

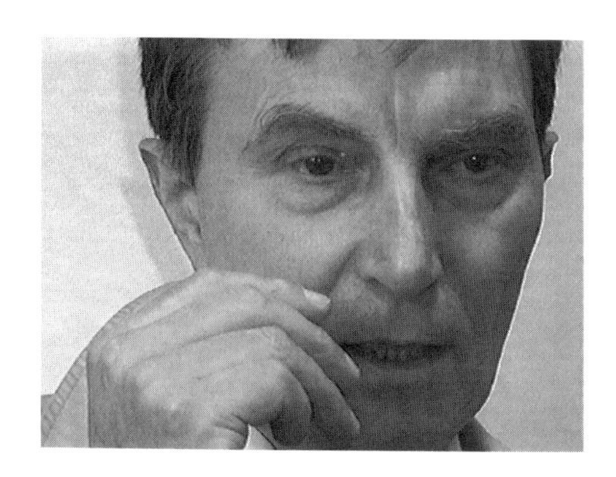

The patient was suffering from **Parkinson's disease**, a condition characterized by tremor, rigidity and bradykinesia.

Parkinson's disease is a progressive degenerative disease of the extrapyramidal motor system caused by destruction of the dopaminergic neurones that project from the substantia nigra to the caudate nucleus and putamen. The characteristic histological finding is the Lewy body. Treatment with levodopa (which replenishes striatal dopamine), together with a dopa decarboxylase inhibitor to limit the peripheral side-effects of the medication, is particularly useful for bradykinesia, but does not influence survival. Other dopaminergic drugs, such as bromocriptine or lisuride, are also useful, but are associated with a high incidence of side-effects. Antimuscarinic drugs are thought to act by decreasing the relative excess of central cholinergic transmission, and are particularly useful for tremor.

Tremor is widespread, but most noticeable in the hands. It is said to occur predominantly at rest. Thus, a cup of tea smoothly raised to the lips is spilt when it arrives there, unlike cerebellar disease where the tea cup is emptied of its contents by intention tremor on its way to the sufferer's lips. The movement of the thumb against the index finger is known as 'pill rolling', as it closely resembles the movement used to hand make pills.

Muscular rigidity during passive flexion and extension of the limbs, with superimposed tremor, produces a ratcheting effect known as cogwheel rigidity.

Bradykinesia, difficulty initiating movement, is responsible for the paucity of facial expression, and is often one of the most troublesome symptoms of the condition. In this patient, the original symptoms of difficulty in shaving and turning over in bed were due to this phenomenon. Patients often find themselves 'stuck to the floor' and, when walking, their posture is similar to that adopted by people pushing a wheelbarrow. If the frequency of swallowing is greatly reduced, the patient may appear to salivate excessively and dribble.

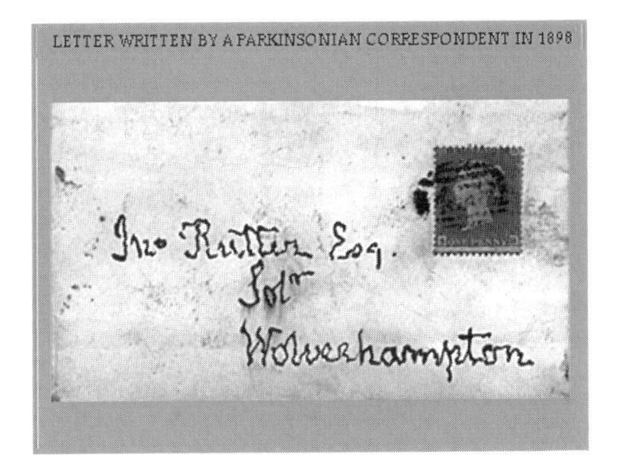

LETTER WRITTEN BY A PARKINSONIAN CORRESPONDENT IN 1898

Reduced facial expressivity is also a feature of depression and, as the two frequently coexist, special care should be taken to elicit symptoms of depressed mood and treat the patients accordingly.

Other features of the condition are on–off attacks. These, as the name suggests, are episodes of rapid, dramatic worsening of bradykinesia that can be extremely troublesome and potentially dangerous. Shy–Drager syndrome is autonomic neuropathy associated with Parkinson's disease.

Basic science

Basal ganglia structure and function

The basal ganglia are paired masses of grey matter, deep to the cerebral cortex, that subserve motor functions distinct from those of the corticospinal (pyramidal) tracts. Defective function of the basal ganglia is responsible for the characteristic movement disorders seen in Parkinson's disease, Huntington's chorea and Wilson's disease. The basal ganglia consist of a cluster of anatomically and, to some extent, functionally distinct groups of nerve cells that receive extensive cholinergic and peptidergic inputs from the brain stem and cortex. Efferents from the basal ganglia are directed to the supplementary motor area and these, together with cerebellar inputs to the primary motor and premotor cortex, control the initiation and coordination of volitional motor acts.

Movement disorders caused by degeneration of the basal ganglia

Akinesia (also bradykinesia and hypokinesia). Refers to difficulty in initiating changes in motor activity, whether in starting a movement or modifying one that is already in progress. The paucity of movement that results is particularly noticeable when the patient attempts to carry out learned motor plans, such as walking, washing, shaving, dressing and so on.

Rigidity. Unlike spasticity caused by lesions of the corticospinal tract, which tends to be minimal until muscles are stretched then diminishes again as full extension approaches (clasp-knife phenomenon), rigidity in extrapyramidal disease is present to the same degree throughout passive movement (lead pipe-like). Tendon reflexes are exaggerated in spastic states, but normal in rigidity caused by basal ganglia disease.

Chorea. Choreic movements (after *khoreia*, 'dance' in Greek) are forcible, rapid, irregular and jerky movements that occur at rest or superimposed on volitional movements. They can affect all motor groups, but may be confined to one side of the body, one limb or restricted to the cranial nerves (i.e. tardive dyskinesia, following chronic neuroleptic administration). Damage to the subthalamic nucleus results in a related condition, hemiballismus, in which violent, flinging movements of the arm occur contralaterally.

Athetosis. Athetosis is the inability to sustain groups of muscles, usually in the limbs, in one position. The result is writhing movements that are slower than those seen in chorea, but may be difficult to distinguish from the latter.

Dystonias. Dystonias are conditions characterized by fixed abnormal twisting postures, frequently involving the trunk rather than the axial muscles, caused by spasmodically increased tone. They increase during volitional movements, particularly when the patient is nervous or stressed, and disappear during sleep.

Myoclonus. This is a very brief, involuntary muscular contraction that occurs at rest, during voluntary movements or in response to sensory stimuli. The opposite, transient loss of tone leading to a brief lapse of posture, is called asterixis.

Tremor. Tremor involves rhythmic oscillating movements of the body about a fixed point, usually involving the hands, but also the feet, head, tongue or jaw.

MCQs

1 Basal ganglia efferents control the initiation and coordination of volitional motor acts.
2 Degeneration of the basal ganglia typically results in muscle weakness.
3 The progression of Parkinson's disease can be halted by appropriate treatment.
4 Dopamine and dopaminergic drugs primarily influence tremor.
5 Clasp-knife rigidity, which varies depending on the extent of flexion of a limb, is characteristic of Parkinson's disease.

Case 35

The man who got into the bath but couldn't get out

History

A 35-year-old company director developed aching retro-orbital discomfort one evening, a few hours before retiring to bed. He awoke the following morning to find himself blind in that eye and, after being referred directly to the emergency department of the local eye hospital by his doctor, a diagnosis of optic neuritis was made. With steroid treatment, he slowly regained peripheral vision over the subsequent 4 months and for a time remained completely well. Some months later, however, while playing football with his sons, he began to notice that when he extended his neck he felt acutely dizzy. Over the following 8 years, he suffered a series of episodes during which his legs became progressively weaker and his coordination gradually worsened. He also noticed that hot weather and particularly hot baths dramatically exacerbated the weakness in his arms and legs, and that flexing his neck produced fleeting, but severe, stabbing pains in his back and neck. On one occasion he recalled finding himself too weak to get out of a hot bath. He had to let the water out and remain in the empty tub for 30 min before his strength had returned sufficiently to allow him to make his escape. As his coordination had worsened, eating had become more difficult, and he confided that consuming soup was impossible.

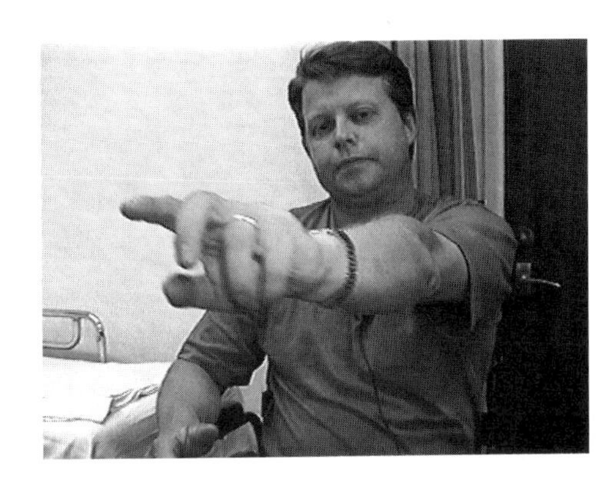

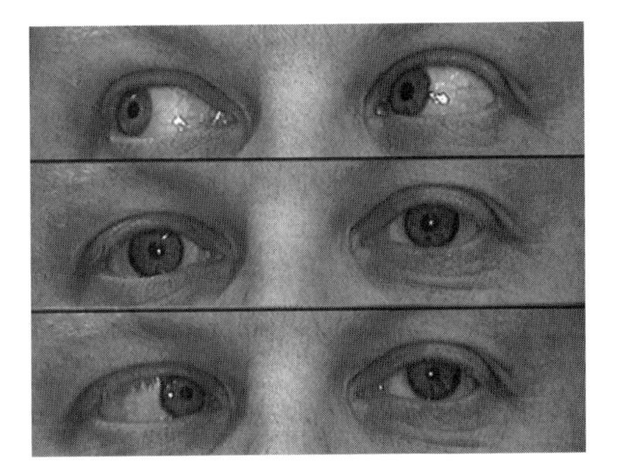

Notes

The patient had multiple sclerosis presenting with optic neuritis.

On examination, he was confined to a wheelchair, but was surprisingly cheerful about his predicament. All of the abnormal findings were related to his nervous system. Finger movements only were visible in the right eye and a large central scotoma was present. **Ataxic nystagmus** was present on testing eye movements, and muscle power was reduced in the upper limbs to three-fifths and in the lower limbs to one-fifth of normal strength. Marked cerebellar signs were present with a coarse intention tremor, past pointing and severe dysdiadochokinesia. Speech was quite normal and higher mental function was preserved.

A magnetic resonance scan of his brain revealed multiple areas of demyelination. Visual evoked responses were slowed (as nerve conduction is impaired in demyelinated fibres), and a sample of cerebrospinal fluid (CSF) obtained subsequently contained slightly raised protein levels but a high immunoglobulin G (IgG) to albumin ratio.

Multiple sclerosis, a condition that affects 1:10 000 people in Northern Europe, is an autoimmune condition, triggered possibly by genetic, infectious or environmental factors, that usually presents with recurrent, random attacks of one or more asymmetrical foci of demyelination in the central nervous system. Demyelination in multiple sclerosis is characterized by the involvement of discrete, well-defined areas, from a few millimetres to several centimetres in diameter, known as plaques, that are scattered throughout the white matter of the brain and spinal cord and extend into the cerebral grey matter (with the preservation of nerve cell bodies). The peripheral nerves are not affected and the plaques in the central nervous system do not conform to anatomical boundaries. Because the plaques may involve relatively non-eloquent areas of the brain, it is estimated that up to 20% of cases of multiple sclerosis do not manifest during life. When it does, the disease tends to begin in early adulthood, with episodes of demyelination that develop over days or months, followed by partial (or even complete) remission before the next episode, which may occur within days or after several decades have passed. In addition to the classical relapsing remitting pattern, one-third of patients develop a chronic progressive form and, in others, the condition appears to stabilize, with no new symptoms occurring even over a long period of time.

Approximately 40% of patients with multiple sclerosis have an episode of optic neuritis. Of those who present with optic neuritis, 40% go on to develop multiple sclerosis. The changes in severity of symptoms with even minor changes in body temperature are characteristic, as is an electric shock-like sensation on flexing the neck (Lhermitte's sign). Spinal cord involvement is a dominant feature of multiple sclerosis and many patients develop transverse myelitis and paraparesis. Extensive involvement of the cerebral hemispheres may occur and, although depression is common (and occurred in this patient), euphoria can also occur.

A combination of brain stem and long tract (pyramidal) signs is typical of multiple sclerosis. Internuclear ophthalmoplegia, brain stem demyelination affecting the medial longitudinal fasciculus (the fibre bundle that connects the IIIrd, IVth and VIth cranial nerve nuclei) leading to 'ataxic nystagmus', is virtually pathognomonic of multiple sclerosis. In the classical form of ataxic nystagmus, demyelination of the medial longitudinal fasciculus occurs between the IVth and VIth nerve nuclei, resulting in the failure of adduction of the right eye on gaze to the left and of the left eye on gaze to the right, with nystagmus of the abducted eye in each case.

Basic science

The cerebellum consists of a series of midline structures and two hemispheres, each containing a central nucleus (the dentate) through which most cerebellar efferent information passes.

Lesions of the midline structures produce severe ataxia, sometimes making it difficult for the patient to sit unsupported. Tumours of the region often cause IVth nerve palsies and obstruct the aqueduct, causing raised intracranial pressure. Lesions in one of the cerebellar hemispheres cause cerebellar signs on that side. Surprisingly, bilateral cerebellar lesions, such as cerebellar degeneration, cause relatively mild bilateral signs with moderate ataxia. Lesions of the cerebellar peduncles—the connections of the cerebellum to the brain stem—produce the most dramatic cerebellar signs of all, as can lesions of the frontopontocerebellar pathway.

Cerebellar signs

1 Ataxia, which is often severe enough to make the patient frightened to stand unsupported.

2 Ataxia of the arms, so that when both are stretched out in front of the patient the

affected limb rises above the level of the normal. Release of downward pressure on the affected arm causes it to fly up out of control.
3 The finger/nose test, in which the patient with eyes open touches his/her nose and then the examiner's finger. If the examiner's finger is moved, the test can be very sensitive. In severe ataxia, care must be taken to prevent the patient poking himself/herself in the eye.
4 In the legs, the patient is asked to place the heel on the top of the tibia of the opposite leg and run it down the shin, and then lift it off and repeat the manoeuvre.
5 Unilateral ataxia indicates a cerebellar lesion on that side. Marked muscle weakness can often give the appearance of impaired cerebellar function on movement and must be taken into account.
6 Failure to be able to rapidly alternate between movements, such as patting the back of one hand with the palm of the other or alternating the palm and back of one hand on the back of the other, is called dysdiadochokinesia.
7 Nystagmus is not always found in cerebellar disease. Reduced tone and reflexes occur, but are difficult to detect. Sudden vomiting without nausea can occur with changes in posture.

MCQs

1 Of patients presenting with optic neuritis, 40% go on to develop multiple sclerosis.
2 Multiple sclerosis is characterized by recurrent, symmetrical foci of demyelination in the brain and spinal cord.
3 Ataxic nystagmus is caused by demyelination in the medial longitudinal fasciculus.
4 Long tract involvement in multiple sclerosis produces an equal mixture of upper and lower motor neurone signs.
5 Damage to a cerebellar hemisphere produces contralateral signs.

Case 36
The man whose face drooped

History

A 68-year-old former factory worker was seen in the outpatient department for unrelated causes 15 years after the sudden onset of right-sided facial weakness. Looking back, he was able to remember the exact time of day that the problem first appeared (2.45 p.m.) and that he had previously been entirely well. The initial symptom was tingling of the right side of the upper lip, 'as if he had been to the dentist'. He explained that he had not suffered any discomfort behind the ear and had no other neurological symptoms or signs at the time of the problem. Initially, the facial weakness was a major problem and, although it had improved with time, recovery had been incomplete. He had received no treatment for the problem at any time.

On examination, he was seen to have right-sided facial weakness affecting both the upper and lower parts of his face.

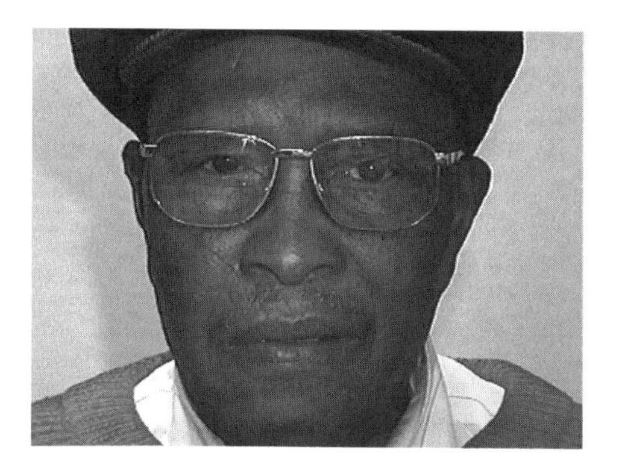

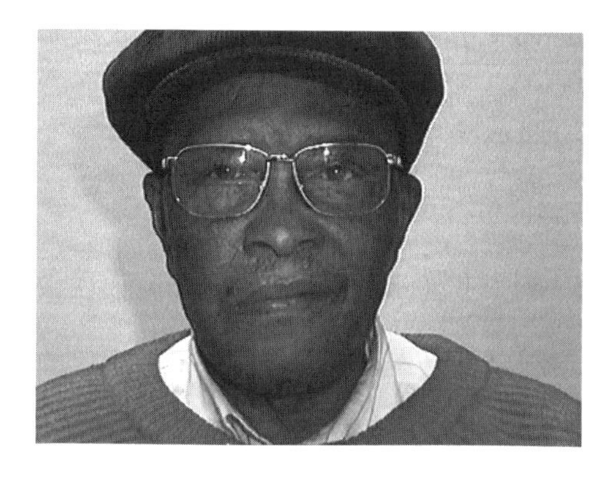

Notes

The patient had Bell's palsy.

Bell's palsy is the most common type of facial palsy with a lifetime incidence of around 1.5%. The pathogenesis is unknown. It is usually characterized by pain behind the ear, followed by the onset of facial weakness that develops over a day or two. Paralysis of the muscles of facial expression frequently leads the patient to describe the affected side of the face as 'numb', although sensory loss is never present on testing. The preservation of some facial movement on the affected side in the first week is a good prognostic sign, and complete recovery occurs in about 60% of patients. One in five patients, however, suffers residual facial weakness with marked asymmetry. A course of prednisolone, 60 mg per day for the first 5 days, is often used but, as the condition is not inflammatory, there is little evidence that it is beneficial. More important is care of the eye, with eyedrops or ointment and protection of the eye at night with padding. The condition is idiopathic, but needs to be distinguished from the Ramsay–Hunt syndrome, infiltration of the VIIth nerve by tumour, compression of the VIIth nerve by an acoustic neuroma, infarcts and tumours that affect the pons and upper medulla. Subtle bilateral facial weakness can occur in Guillain–Barré syndrome and sarcoidosis (uveoparotid fever (Heerfordt's syndrome)).

Table 36.1 Lower motor neurone facial nerve palsy

Site	Signs	Causes
Brain stem	Associated abducent (VIth nerve) palsy and long tract signs. Taste is usually spared	Brain stem stroke, demyelination or glioma
Cerebellopontine angle	Associated trigeminal nerve (Vth nerve) and vestibulocochlear (VIIIth nerve) palsy, with loss of corneal reflex (Vth), deafness and ataxia (VIIIth)	Acoustic neuroma, glioma or other tumour
Facial canal	Lower motor neurone palsy sometimes with pain behind the ear ± hyperacusis and altered taste sensation, but without the above	Bell's palsy, herpes zoster infection, trauma
Distal to facial canal (peripheral nerve)	Lower motor neurone palsy without altered taste or hearing. Parotid enlargement or signs of trauma may be present	Parotid tumour or facial trauma
Muscles of facial expression	Bilateral signs of muscular or neuromuscular pathology may be present	Muscular dystrophy, myasthenia gravis, myotonic dystrophy

Basic science

The facial nerve innervates the muscles of facial expression (tested by asking the patient to screw up the eyes, frown or wrinkle the forehead, smile, purse the lips or blow out the cheeks). Innervation to the upper facial muscles (the muscles of the forehead and those closing the eyes) is bilateral. Lower facial muscle innervation is contralateral. The sensory and secretomotor part of the facial nerve runs adjacent to the motor fibres, but is contained within a separate sheath. It is responsible for innervating the lacrimal and salivary glands, for taste sensation in the anterior two-thirds of the tongue and for a small patch of skin innervation to the ear and the area just behind it that is thought to account for discomfort behind the ear in some cases of Bell's palsy. In upper motor neurone facial nerve lesions, hand and arm weakness is usually present and, if the dominant hemisphere is affected, dysphasia may also be present. In lower motor neurone facial palsy, sounds may seem excessively loud owing to paralysis of the stapedius muscle (hyperacusis), and taste may be affected.

MCQs

1 Areas of facial sensory loss are typically found in Bell's palsy.
2 Between 90 and 95% of patients recover fully from Bell's palsy.
3 Facial nerve paralysis should be included as part of the differential diagnosis of ptosis.
4 The facial nerve subserves touch and taste sensation to the anterior two-thirds of the tongue.
5 In some cases of Bell's palsy, sounds may seem inappropriately loud.

Case 37
Transient right-sided weakness

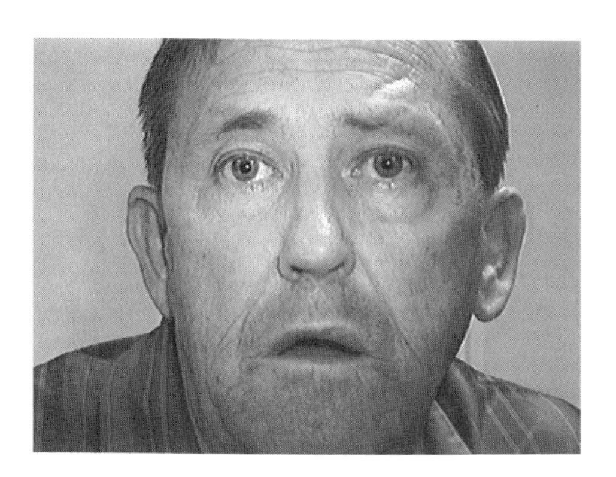

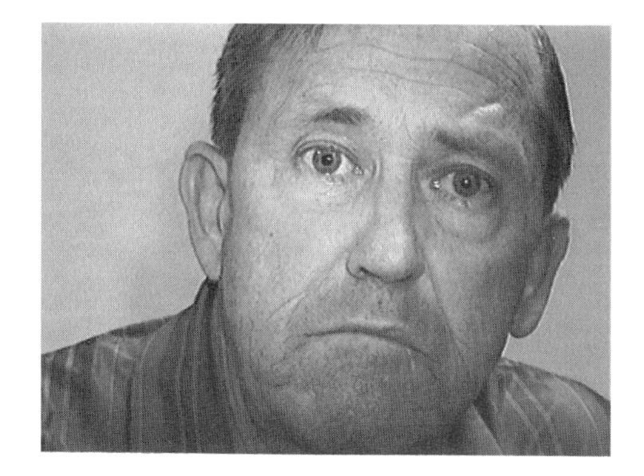

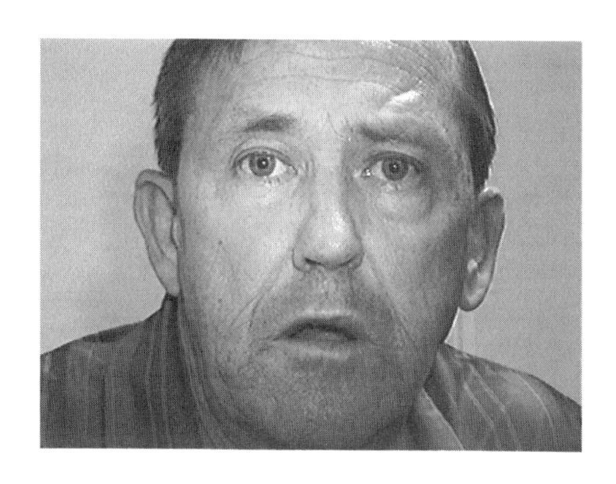

History

A 67-year-old lorry driver was admitted to hospital following a brief episode of weakness, numbness and pins and needles in his right arm and the right side of his body. He had suffered a similar episode 2 years previously from which he had made a full recovery over a period of an hour or two. On this occasion, the paraesthesia was associated with disturbance of his speech and transient double vision. From the age of 20 years until 13 years previously he had smoked up to 60 cigarettes daily, and for much of his driving career his cargo had been sacks of raw asbestos fibres.

He had a past history of a left pneumonectomy for a bronchogenic neoplasm and claimed that 'traces of TB' were found on histological examination of the lung biopsy specimen. From that time on, he had noted breathlessness on exertion, and suffered increasingly frequent episodes of productive cough requiring inpatient antibiotic treatment. He had a past history of febrile convulsions as a child and a splenectomy following a road traffic accident.

The findings on examination were in keeping with his history. In addition to being weak, he was hyporeflexic on the right side and had bilateral downgoing plantar responses. Minimal left-sided signs of Horner's syndrome were also noted. His blood pressure was 172/94 mmHg with a regular pulse of 72 beats per minute. The day after admission his weakness had completely resolved.

Notes

The patient had suffered a transient ischaemic attack (TIA).

A TIA is the abrupt loss of focal cerebral or monocular function presumed to be due to embolic or thrombotic vascular disease, with symptoms lasting less than 24 h. A TIA is associated with a sevenfold increased risk of stroke over the subsequent 5 years, and a 2–3% annual risk of myocardial infarction. The combined risk of vascular death after a TIA is 9% over the first year, with the greatest risk being in the first 3 months, and then about 6% per year for the next 5 years.

Symptoms are sudden in onset, maximum at the outset and often consist of weakness of the whole or part of one side of the body, with numbness rather than tingling if sensory symptoms are evident. Loss of consciousness, dizziness and light-headedness are highly atypical.

The *carotid territory* is affected in 80% of TIAs, producing:

- unilateral weakness or sensory loss,
- monocular visual loss, or
- aphasia.

TIAs in the *vertebrobasilar territory* cause:

- bilateral or alternating weakness,
- sensory loss,
- visual loss,
- dysphagia,
- diplopia,
- dysarthria,
- vertigo, or
- ataxia.

Thromboembolic complications from atherosclerosis of arteries leading to the brain, or within the brain, account for 70% of TIAs. Emboli from the heart are thought to account for 20% of TIAs.

In patients who suffer a TIA, retinal infarction or non-disabling ischaemic stroke, and who have 70–99% carotid artery stenosis, expert carotid surgery confers an eightfold reduction in ipsilateral ischaemic stroke rate (8% to 1%) at 3 years, compared with optimal medical treatment with aspirin, cessation of smoking and control of hypertension and hyperlipidaemia alone.

Basic science

As cessation of cerebral circulation results in unconsciousness within 10 s, it is clear that the brain needs a continuous supply of oxygenated blood on a moment-to-moment basis. Ischaemia for longer than 3 min under normal circumstances causes infarction, with loss of cell membrane integrity and disruption of the blood–brain barrier. The affected grey matter is initially pale, but can subsequently become engorged with petechial haemorrhages and dilated blood vessels. The extent to which the glial fibrotic reaction that results is responsible for making the changes that occur irreversible is currently being challenged and, during the next decade, active management of stroke to minimize such damage may become a reality.

Brain stem ischaemia

Vascular lesions of the brain stem generally produce a defined area of damage in an identifiable vascular territory, and produce symptoms such as diplopia, dysarthria, nausea, vomiting and vertigo.

For the interested reader, these include the following defined areas:

Dorsolateral midbrain infarction. This causes an ipsilateral Horner's syndrome and total loss of sensation on the opposite side. If the superior cerebellar peduncle is damaged, there will also be cerebellar signs on the same side—with tremor, past pointing, inability to perform rapid repeated movements and ataxia.

Paramedian midbrain infarction. Damage to the IIIrd nerve fascicle (i.e. the IIIrd nerve before it emerges from the brain stem) produces a complete IIIrd nerve palsy. The IIIrd nerve nucleus runs over a considerable vertical distance and may be partially damaged.

Damage to the red nucleus causes marked cerebellar signs in the limbs on the opposite side.

Basal midbrain infarction. Damage to the IIIrd nerve fascicle produces a complete IIIrd nerve palsy. Infarction of the corticospinal bundles produces hemiplegia of the contralateral limbs and face.

Dorsolateral pontine infarction This causes an ipsilateral Horner's syndrome with loss of pain and temperature sensation on the opposite side of the body. In lower pontine lesions, the Vth nerve may be involved, causing ipsilateral facial numbness, and, lower still, involvement of the VIIIth nerve nucleus causes vertigo, nystagmus and deafness as well.

Paramedian pontine infarction. This is the level of the VIth nerve nucleus. As connections to the IIIrd nerve are also damaged, conjugate movements (i.e. gaze to the side of the lesion) are interrupted. As the VIIth nerve fascicle wraps around the VIth nerve nucleus, an ipsilateral VIIth nerve palsy (Bell's palsy) also occurs, sometimes with loss of touch and proprioception to the opposite side of the body (if the medial lemniscus is involved).

Basal pontine infarction. Contralateral hemiplegia occurs with ipsilateral lower motor neurone VIth and VIIth nerve lesions. With a discrete lesion, the only signs may be a VIth nerve palsy with weakness of the opposite arm.

Dorsolateral infarction of the medulla. This produces Wallenberg's syndrome, characterized by Horner's syndrome, ipsilateral Vth nerve palsy with loss of sensation over the face and loss of pain and temperature sensation on the opposite side of the body. The lower part of the VIIIth nerve nuclei and the cerebellar peduncles are involved, producing severe vertigo, nystagmus, nausea, vomiting and ipsilateral ataxia. Involvement of the IXth and Xth nerves causes dysphagia and sometimes hiccoughs.

Paramedian and basal infarction of the medulla. In the medulla, bilateral infarction may occur producing the 'locked-in' syndrome, in which the fully conscious patient with globally impaired sensation cannot move or speak. Unilateral infarction produces a XIIth nerve lesion with contralateral hemiplegia and loss of fine touch and proprioception.

MCQs

1 A TIA is associated with a sevenfold increased risk of stroke over the subsequent 5 years.
2 TIA is part of the differential diagnosis of transient loss of consciousness.
3 Most TIAs affect the vertebrobasilar territory.
4 In TIA associated with a 90% carotid artery stenosis, carotid surgery increases survival over 3 months.
5 Infarction of the paramedian and basal (anterior) brain stem produces Horner's syndrome.

Case 38
Unilateral weakness after a headache

History

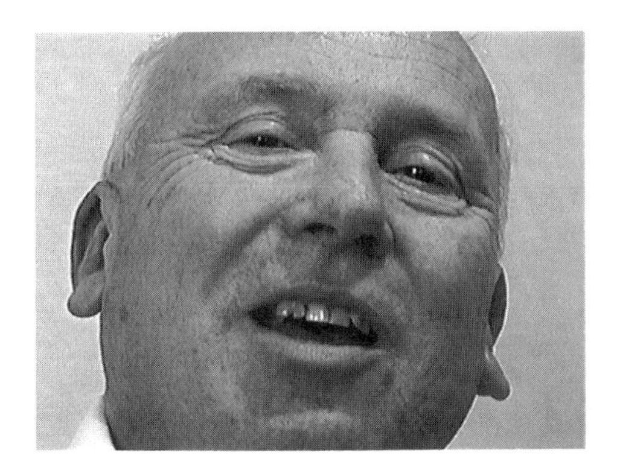

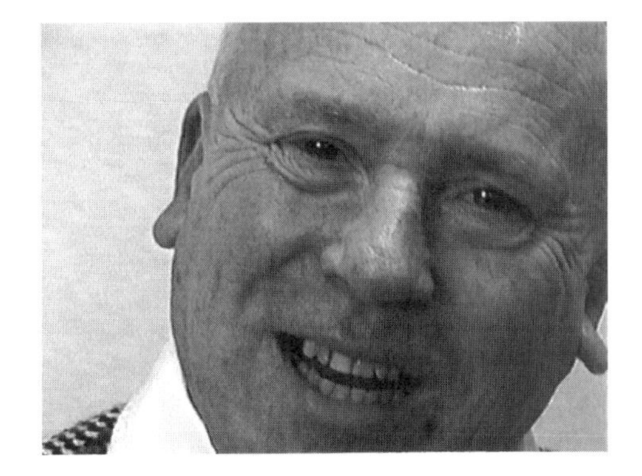

A 43-year-old company director with no previous contact with the medical profession found, on waking on the morning of admission, that he was unable to move his right arm or leg. He had suffered from a mild frontal headache the night before, but denied any sensory abnormalities in his limbs either before or after the onset of weakness. He was a non-smoker and drank alcohol in moderation.

On initial examination, his blood pressure was 204/110 mmHg. He was slightly drowsy, with a right-sided flaccid hemiparesis, absent reflexes and an absent plantar response on that side. Several hours later he was re-examined and was found to be hypertonic on the right side with increased tendon reflexes and an upgoing plantar response. Sensation, visual fields, comprehension and ability to communicate were preserved.

His fasting blood glucose level was 5.6 mmol L^{-1} with an HbA1c of 5%. His total cholesterol level was 5 mmol L^{-1} (192 mg dL^{-1}), syphilis serology was negative and a computerized tomography (CT) scan of his head on the day of admission showed no abnormalities. Some flexion power in his arm and extension power of his legs returned over the following 6 months and remained stable thereafter.

Notes

The patient had suffered a left-sided cerebrovascular accident (with right-sided signs) that is likely to have involved a lenticulostriate branch of the left middle cerebral artery and the posterior limb of the internal capsule it supplied (see figure on page 105).

Sensory and motor fibres running between the cortex and brain stem form the corona radiata, a fan-shaped bundle that becomes the internal capsule as it is compressed between the lentiform nucleus which indents it laterally and the thalamus and head of the caudate nucleus which compress it medially at either end. The blood supply to the internal capsule is derived from six to eight small, perforating branches of the middle cerebral artery called the lenticulostriate arteries.

It is likely that temporary occlusion of one or more lenticulostriate arteries was responsible for this patient's stroke. The vessels frequently recanalize after irreversible damage has been done and the lesions are often too small to be seen on CT scan.

Worldwide the prevalence of stroke is about 0.5%, with an 8–20% mortality within the first month. The overall 5-year survival rate is 60% for women and 55% for men, with 60% of survivors in both sexes having significant disability. In Europe, the incidence of stroke is ≈0.2%. Of these, 80% are ischaemic and 20% haemorrhagic. Of the ischaemic strokes, only 17% are related directly to carotid artery pathology and, of these, the usual pathology is atherosclerosis at the carotid bifurcation, which narrows the vessel and promotes the formation of thrombotic fragments which embolize into the brain.

Risk factors for stroke are:

- increasing age,
- hypertension,
- smoking,
- diabetes mellitus, and
- hyperlipidaemia.

Evidence of vascular disease in other parts of the body, such as ischaemic heart disease, claudication and aortic aneurysm, is also frequently present.

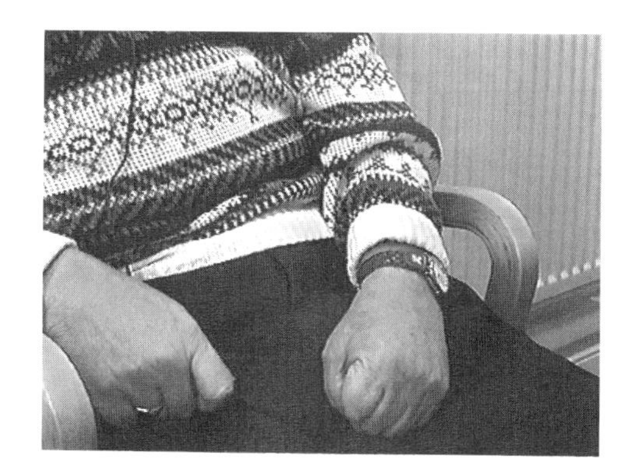

Basic science

Vascular territories within the cerebral hemispheres

Anterior cerebral artery occlusion. This causes flaccid paralysis of the leg (even though the lesion is upper motor neurone, as cortical control is lost) with cortical sensory loss (i.e. affects touch and proprioception) and urinary incontinence. In some instances, the arm is affected by a spastic paralysis, and there is damage to memory and intellect. Occlusion of the perforating branch is very rare, but produces weakness of the face and arm without dysphasia. Occlusion of the terminal branch produces flaccid weakness of the leg with brisk reflexes and an extensor plantar response.

Middle cerebral artery occlusion. Occlusion of the main trunk causes massive infarction of the hemisphere, often associated with oedema-induced coma. Hemianaesthesia and a complete homonymous hemianopia occur. If the dominant hemisphere is affected, dysphasia results. If the non-dominant hemisphere is affected, dyspraxia or complete denial of the existence of the affected (usually left) side occurs. Pyramidal and extrapyramidal mechanisms are destroyed, so that the weakness is flaccid with little chance of recovery. Occlusion of a carotid artery can cause a similar picture.

Occlusion of a perforating branch of the middle cerebral artery is one of the most frequent vascular catastrophes seen (as occurred in this patient). Both contralateral limbs are affected, resulting in a flaccid hemiparesis. After some hours, tone starts to return, the reflexes become brisk and an extensor plantar response develops. Arm flexor and leg extensor power returns to some extent, giving the classical hemiplegic picture. Sensory deficits and hemianopia are unusual and bad prognostic signs. Dysphasia does not occur because the parietal cortex is not affected.

Occlusion of the terminal branch of the middle cerebral artery causes either mild or profound inability to speak or comprehend speech, sometimes associated with flaccid paralysis of the face and arm.

Posterior cerebral artery occlusion. Occlusion of the main trunk causes variable degrees of confusion and memory deficit, although

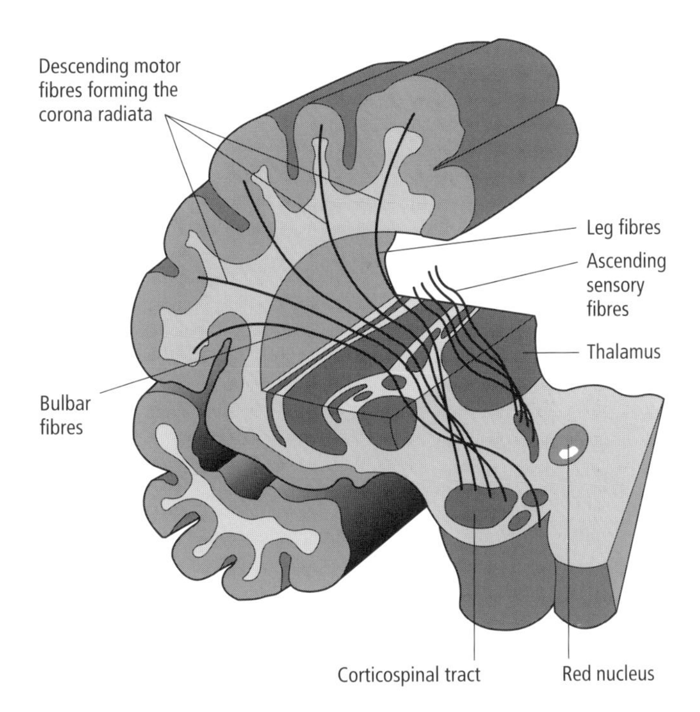

Adapted with permission from *Neurological Differential Diagnosis*, 2nd Edn, J.P. Patten, 1996. © Springer-Verlag.

these symptoms are more typical of bilateral damage caused by occlusion of the basilar artery. There may be sensory and visual deficits, depending on the pattern of anastomoses.

Occlusion of a perforating branch causes complete hemianopia and hemianaesthesia which can become severe hyperaesthesia. Hemiballismus, wild, unilateral flinging movements of the limbs, may occur if the upper brain stem is affected. This is the only extrapyramidal syndrome typically produced by vascular disease. Occlusion of a terminal branch causes macular sparing hemianopia, which quite often accompanies migraine in young otherwise fit people.

MCQs

1 Eighty per cent of strokes are ischaemic rather than haemorrhagic.
2 Hypercholesterolaemia is a risk factor for stroke.
3 Dysphasia suggests damage to the non-dominant hemisphere.
4 Hemiplegia, hemianaesthesia and hemianopia are characteristic of middle cerebral artery occlusion.
5 Posterior cerebral artery occlusion characteristically produces cerebellar signs.

Case 39
A painful rash and aching ankles

History

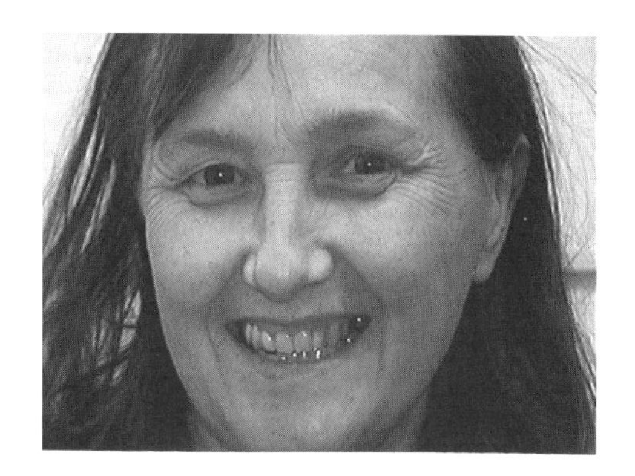

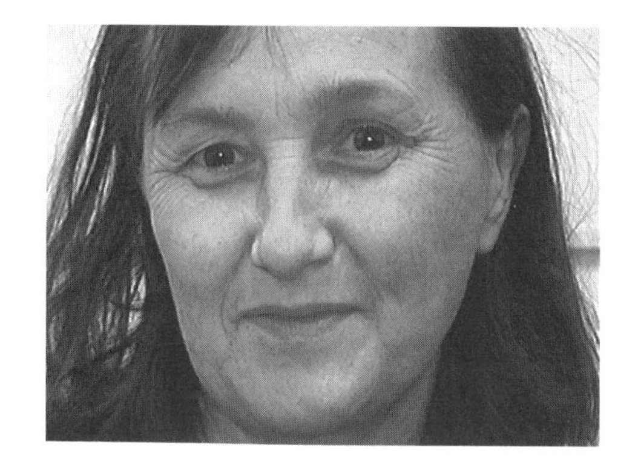

A 50-year-old physiotherapist was admitted with a 2-day history of a rash and arthralgia. Apart from a tooth extraction the previous week, she had previously been entirely well. The problem started as a series of raised, red patches on her legs, thighs and ankles which she initially took to be insect bites. The day after their first appearance, however, the onset of discomfort on movement of her left ankle, followed hours later by pain on movement of the right ankle, suggested a more complex pathology. She presented to her doctor who referred her to hospital.

The patient had not been abroad but, in the course of her job, had experienced contact with many 'ill' people. She had no history of inflammatory bowel disease and had not had any symptoms of a chest infection. After a very positive reaction to a Heaf test as a child, she had undergone a series of chest X-rays at intervals that excluded active tuberculosis (TB).

Notes

The patient had erythema nodosum.

Erythema nodosum is a form of panniculitis (inflammation of the subcuticular fat) seen most commonly in young women. The bilateral, sometimes exquisitely tender, red nodules on the anterior surface of the legs, and sometimes on the thighs, forearms or even face, are accompanied by arthralgia, fever and sometimes joint swelling. The condition often occurs in isolation, as it did in this case, but can be associated with:

- inflammatory bowel disease,
- sarcoidosis,
- treatment with sulphonamides,
- TB, or
- a streptococcal infection.

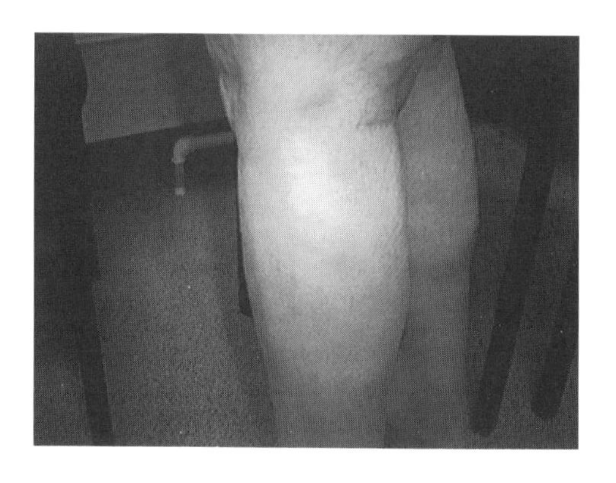

Sarcoidosis involves the skin in 25% of cases, and the most frequent lesion is erythema nodosum, although plaques, maculopapular eruptions, subcutaneous nodules and lupus pernio are also common.

The lesions of erythema nodosum usually feel as if they are deep to the skin rather than in it, and are usually 5–20 mm in diameter with ill-defined margins. Recurrent crops of lesions may develop over days or months, but in most cases the lesions resolve within 2 weeks. The erythrocyte sedimentation rate is usually raised.

Basic science

Fat

Unlike other types of cells that contain very little fat, adipocytes, the cellular elements of adipose tissue, are almost entirely fat filled. Adipocytes are found predominantly subcutaneously and in the abdominal cavity. As fats are highly reduced, their energy density is more than double that of protein or carbohydrate, and the 21–26% fat content of normal humans provides enough energy to withstand starvation for 2 or 3 months. The reason for this is not only that the fats are highly reduced, but that they are very non-polar and can be stored in an almost anhydrous form. Humans lack the enzymes to introduce double bonds distal to C-9 in fatty acids, and therefore require dietary linoleate and linolenate, the latter being the key precursor of prostaglandins and other signal molecules. There is no dietary requirement for cholesterol.

In addition to their function as an energy store and the thermal insulating effect of subcutaneous fat, fatty acids are the building blocks of phospholipids and glycolipids, and serve as hormones and intracellular second messengers. Fat is also endocrinologically active, as the enzyme aromatase that it contains is responsible for converting preandrogens, such as dehydroxyepiandrosterone and androstenedione, to testosterone, or to the cyclic oestrogen 'oestrone'. By stimulating luteinizing hormone release from the pituitary gland, oestrone stimulates ovarian production of preandrogens, and further peripheral conversion of circulating preandrogens by adipose tissue results in an increase in effective androgen levels.

Brown adipose tissue, like white adipose tissue, contains large amounts of triglycerides. The brown colour of brown adipose tissue is caused by the cytochrome content of the numerous mitochondria that it contains, each of which, in turn, contains relatively large amounts of the protein thermogenin on the inner membranes. In brown fat, energy derived from oxidation is released as heat rather than stored as high energy phosphate bonds. This thermogenic activity, derived from the uncoupling of electron transport from oxidative phosphorylation, is stimulated principally through its dense sympathetic innervation and, to a lesser extent, by an increase in circulating levels of noradrenaline. The action of noradrenaline (norepinephrine) on hormone-sensitive triacylglycerol lipase cleaves triglycerides into glycerol and fatty acids within adipose tissue, and thermogenesis is activated by the latter.

MCQs

1 Erythema nodosum is a form of inflammation of the fat.
2 Fats are energy dense owing to their highly oxidized state.
3 The average fat content of the body is sufficient to supply energy needs for up to a week.
4 Adipose tissue contains the enzyme 5α-reductase.
5 The dietary requirement for cholesterol is similar to that of the essential fatty acids.

Case 40
Aching muscles and morning stiffness

History

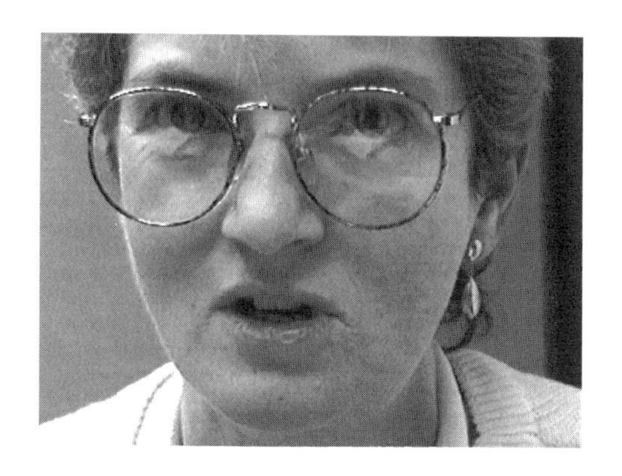

A 45-year-old woman, previously completely well, presented to her doctor with a 1-week history of discomfort and swelling in the hands and fingers. This was more noticeable first thing in the morning and eased off during the day. She also felt generally unwell, with aching in the muscles, anorexia and tiredness, and was woken at night by tingling in the fingers. With the exception of the arthritis identified by the patient, there were no abnormal findings on examination, and she denied any pain in her shoulders or knees, but did complain of some foot discomfort when weight bearing. She had not suffered from jaundice, psoriasis or gout, and had not had any backache. Over the subsequent few weeks, the fever subsided and, aided by non-steroidal anti-inflammatory drugs, the acute joint pain abated. Other joints, particularly her wrists, knees and shoulders, were affected over the ensuing months, however, and she noticed the gradual development of deformities in her hands and the appearance of non-tender, hard, subcutaneous nodules at her wrists and elbows.

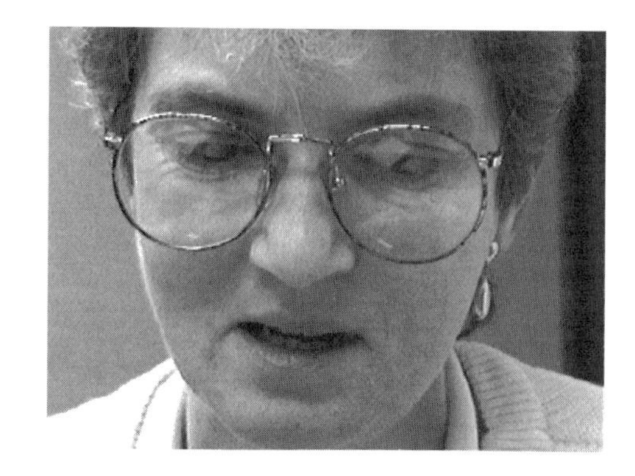

Notes

The patient had **rheumatoid arthritis** and was found to be rheumatoid factor positive.

Rheumatoid arthritis is a persistent, peripheral, symmetrical polyarthritis that affects around 3% of the population and tends to occur more in women than men. Synovial inflammation and enlargement spreads over the joint cartilage as 'pannus', which appears to contribute to the destruction of the underlying cartilage and bone. The result is *swelling, warmth and tenderness of affected joints and tendon sheaths.*

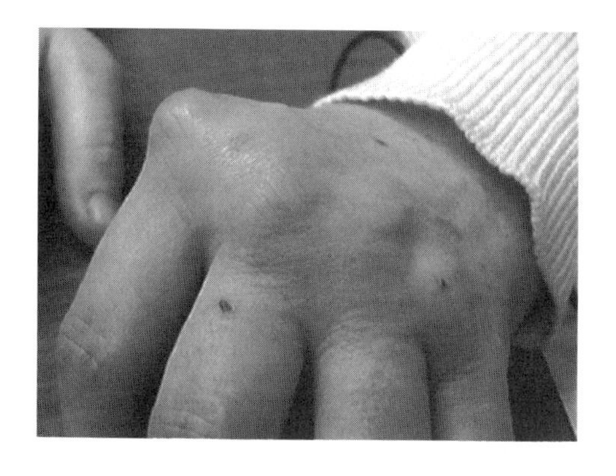

Swelling between the knuckles and fingers makes it difficult for the patient to make a fist or to fully extend the fingers. *Swollen toes and knees* are also typical findings, and *destruction of cartilage and bone, stretching, dislocation and rupture of tendons and subluxation and dislocation of joints lead to the characteristic deformities* which include ulnar deviation of the fingers, swan-neck and *boutonnière* deformities, 'Z' deformity of the thumbs, subluxation of the metacarpophalangeal joints and ruptured extensor tendons. In this patient, swelling around the wrist also produced *carpal tunnel syndrome* with tingling and discomfort in the hands and forearms during the night. *Rheumatoid nodules*, firm, round, non-tender nodules usually found at pressure points, such as the elbows, Achilles tendon and sacrum, occur in around 25% of patients. Heterogeneous immunoglobulin M (IgM), IgG and IgA antibodies specific for the Fc fragment of IgG are known as '*rheumatoid factors*', and over 50% of patients have the histocompatibility antigen HLA-DW4.

Extra-articular features of rheumatoid disease include anaemia (often normochromic, normocytic), nodule formation, muscle wasting, lymphadenopathy, peripheral oedema, episcleritis, Sjögren's syndrome (keratoconjunctivitis sicca and xerostomia), nail-fold vasculitis, peripheral sensory neuropathy, pleural and pericardial effusions, pulmonary fibrosis, systemic vasculitis, splenomegaly and periarticular osteoporosis.

Basic science

Joints are either fibrous, cartilaginous or synovial.

Fibrous joints occur as sutures (found only between the bones that form the skull) that fuse in adulthood to form synostoses. Syndesmoses are fibrous joints in which the bones are joined by fibrous tissue ligaments that allow a jog of movement or limited rotation, such as the distal end of the tibia and fibula and the slightly more mobile fibrous connection between the ulna and radius. The third type of fibrous joint is the gomphosis, characterized by the joint between a tooth and its alveolar socket, held in place by the short periodontal ligaments.

Cartilaginous joints, in contrast, unite bones with a cartilaginous plate that provides the sites of bone growth during youth, but is obliterated by fusion at the end of puberty. A typical example is an epiphyseal plate that connects the diaphysis (shaft) and epiphysis of a long bone. The symphysis joints of the intervertebral discs are further examples of cartilaginous joints.

Synovial joints are characterized by a joint cavity lined either side by cartilaginous articular surfaces. The joint is surrounded by an articular capsule, filled with synovial fluid, which has a viscous consistency resulting from its hyaluronic acid content, and reinforced by ligaments that may be inside the capsule, exterior to the capsule or form part of the capsule itself.

MCQs

1 Rheumatoid arthritis is closely associated with the HLA-B27 antigen.
2 Heberden's nodes are associated with rheumatoid arthritis.
3 Rheumatoid arthritis is associated with sight-threatening eye inflammation.
4 Sutures, syndesmoses and gomphoses are types of fibrous joint.
5 The synovial joints that join the shafts and epiphyses of long bones fuse at puberty.

Case 41
Episodic joint pains

History

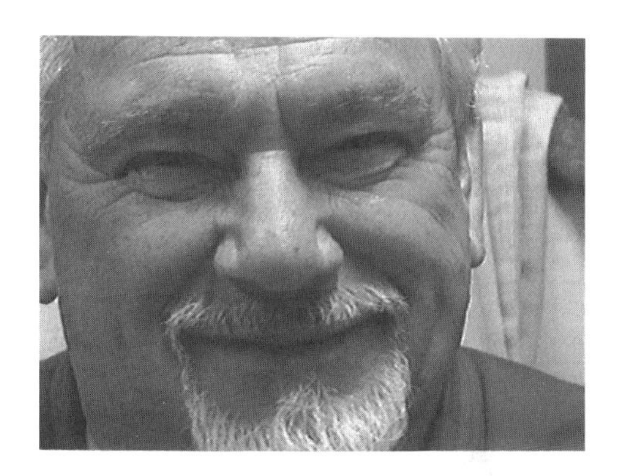

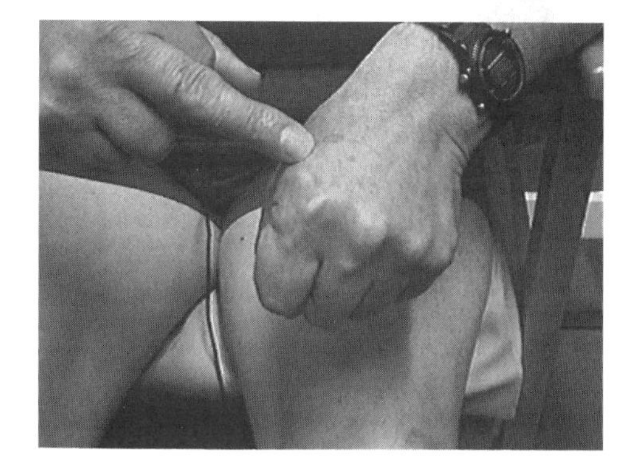

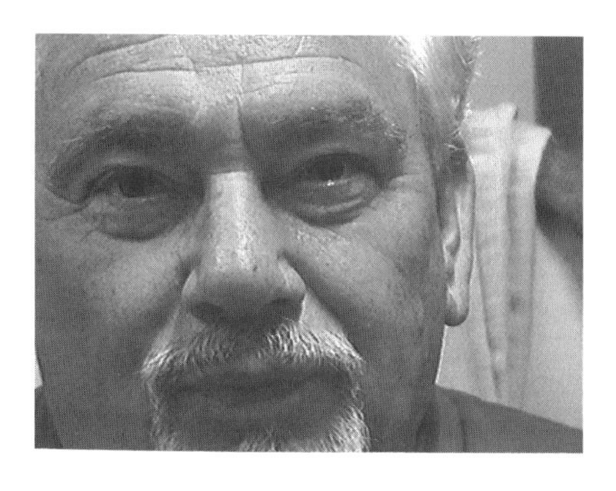

A 57-year-old man was seen in clinic with a long history of episodes of arthritis in his knees, elbows, interphalangeal, metacarpophalangeal and metatarsophalangeal joints. The history had started with an acutely swollen knee at the age of 38 years, which had been treated with steroids, analgesics and physiotherapy. He had not injured the joint, and had no history of sexual intercourse with a new partner. Joint aspiration had revealed negatively birefringent crystals, and a diagnosis of acute gout had been made. The swelling took several weeks to subside, but, at intervals of several weeks to several months over the following years, further exquisitely painful attacks of seemingly spontaneous inflammation affected his knees, elbows and the small joints of his hands and feet asymmetrically. Each attack was treated with anti-inflammatories and colchicine. As time passed, he noticed that a series of small swellings over the extensor tendons of his fingers and the metacarpophalangeal joints had developed. There was no history of renal colic or renal impairment, and he had no family history of gout.

At the time of examination he was asymptomatic, but tophi were present over the extensor tendons of his fingers and the metacarpophalangeal joints. Serum levels of urate and his urea and electrolytes were within normal limits.

Notes

The patient had gout.

The full manifestations of gout include:

- an increase in serum urate (at some time),
- recurrent attacks of acute arthritis caused

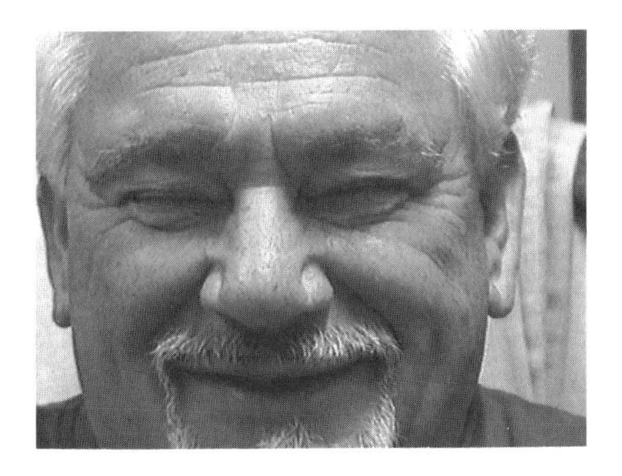

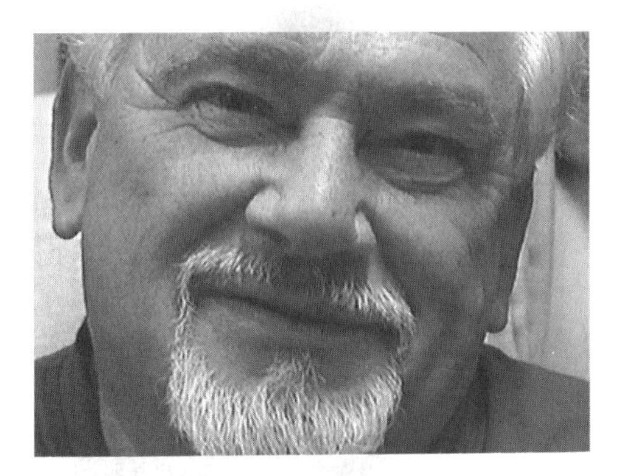

by precipitation of sodium urate crystals in synovial fluid, and
- tophi—aggregations of sodium urate crystals in soft tissues, such as the antihelix of the ear and Achilles tendon, and around the peripheral joints, causing pain and deformity.

Uric acid nephrolithiasis and direct interstitial renal damage are also typical of the condition. Before dialysis became available, up to 25% of patients with gouty arthritis died in renal failure.

As renal failure causes hyperuricaemia, it can be difficult to tell whether hyperuricaemia in patients with chronic renal failure is the cause or the result of the condition.

Basic science

Hyperuricaemia

Humans have no dietary requirement for purines. The intestinal mucosa oxidizes dietary purines (in nucleic acids, adenosine triphosphate (ATP), cyclic adenosine monophosphate (cAMP) and cyclic guanosine

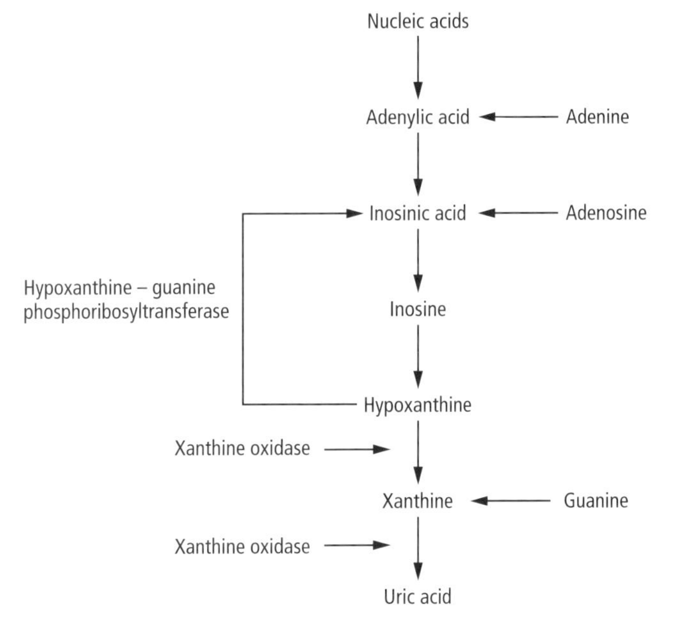

monophosphate (cGMP)) to **uric acid** which, compared with allantoin produced by many other species, is extremely insoluble (7 mg per 100 mL of serum at 37 °C). Almost all of the manifestations of gout result directly or indirectly from the formation of sodium urate crystals in synovial fluid, leading to the development of acute synovitis. Any joint of the body can be affected either singly or together, with the first metatarsophalangeal joint most often the first involved.

The association between gout and circulating uric acid levels is relatively poor, and fewer than 5% of patients with hyperuricaemia develop gout. Nevertheless, gout only occurs in patients who are, or who have been, hyperuricaemic.

Secondary gout is related to increased purine turnover in haematological conditions, such as polycythaemia, and to massive cellular breakdown following radiotherapy or chemotherapy. Diuretic treatment is an important precipitant of acute gout through decreased renal uric acid clearance.

Renal stones are commonly associated with hyperuricaemia. Up to 40% of patients with hyperuricaemia experience an episode of renal colic before they have their first attack of gout, and many patients with gout have some degree of renal impairment.

A number of rare genetic diseases are also associated with hyperuricaemia. These include xanthinuria, familial juvenile hyperuricaemic nephropathy, phosphoribosylpyrophosphate superactivity, hereditary orotic aciduria and Lesch–Nyhan syndrome, which results from a deficiency of hypoxanthine-guanine phosphoribosyltransferase.

MCQs

1 The tendency to hyperuricaemia is familial.
2 Patients with gout have persistent hyperuricaemia.
3 Microscopy of aspirate from an acute inflamed gouty joint typically reveals negatively birefringent crystals under polarized light.
4 Gout is more common in obese persons.
5 Up to 90% of patients with gout have an attack involving the great toe at some time.

Case 42
Tiredness, aching joints and erectile dysfunction

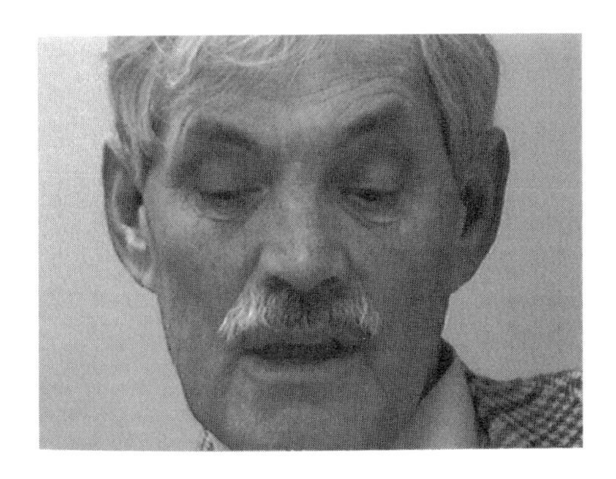

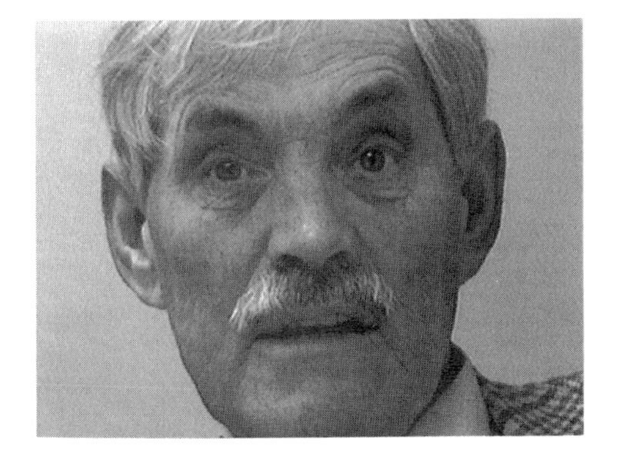

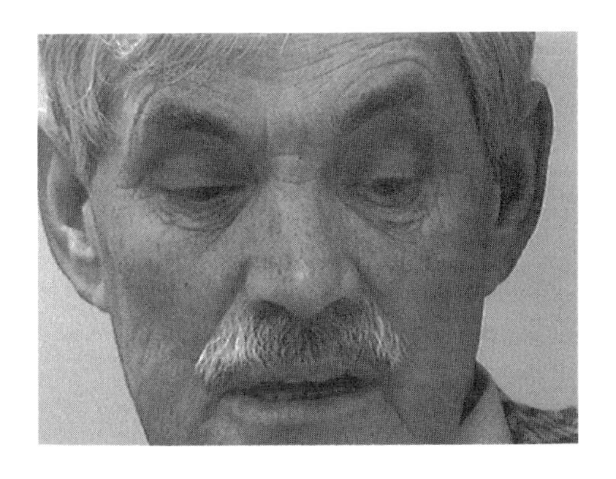

History

A 57-year-old man presented with a 6-month history of lethargy and aching joints. He had been a veterinary surgeon, previously in good health, who, on a number of occasions over the previous 3 months, had presented to his doctor with various complaints of tiredness, lethargy, abdominal discomfort and aching joints, particularly his hands and knees. Each time, the doctor noted that the patient looked tanned and well, and having considered but excluded diagnoses of brucellosis, rheumatoid arthritis, osteoarthritis and depression, had offered reassurance only. On the latest occasion, however, a careful examination was undertaken, and a 3 cm liver edge prompted referral of the patient for a second opinion.

Further history in clinic revealed that the patient drank alcohol in moderation, had not suffered from or been exposed to anyone with hepatitis, had not had any transfusions or other parenteral intervention and had not recently travelled abroad. These was no evidence of jaundice, anaemia, lymphadenopathy, spider naevi or bruising on examination and, in keeping with his doctor's findings, a 4-cm, non-tender, smooth liver edge was palpable on abdominal examination. The spleen was impalpable, but the patient was noted to have mild gynaecomastia and small, soft testes. It was also clear that he had lost most of his axillary and pubic hair, and had noticed that his scalp hair had become more 'silky' and that the distribution of fat on his body had changed to a less masculine pattern.

Asked specifically about erectile function and shaving, he explained that he had not had a spontaneous erection for as long as he could remember, but had not complained to his doctor because he had been widowed 5 years previously and had no particular desire to find a sexual partner. He shaved his beard once every 2–3 days only.

A number of blood tests were undertaken. His HbA1c and fasting blood glucose levels were normal, and he was found to be immune to hepatitis A and B. His ferritin level, however, was grossly elevated at 2300 ng mL^{-1} (normal range, men = 15–400 ng mL^{-1}).

Notes

The patient had haemochromatosis.

Haemochromatosis is an autosomal recessive condition with a carrier (heterozygote) frequency as high as 10% in the general population and a disease frequency of around 1 : 300. Penetrance (physical expression) of the disease is 10 times more common in males, perhaps because of the moderating influence of menstrual- and pregnancy-induced blood loss.

The characteristic *skin pigmentation* is caused by melanin rather than iron and gives rise to the term 'bronze diabetes' for the condition, although the association with diabetes mellitus, caused by pancreatic infiltration, has been challenged. About 50% of patients suffer from *progressive polyarthropathy* and, untreated, deposition of iron in the myocardium produces *dysrhythmias or cardiac failure* in one-third. *Hypogonadism* is caused by iron deposition in the testes and pituitary gland. In this patient, it was this that was responsible, at least in part, for his lethargy, loss of libido and mild gynaecomastia.

At least 80% of cases of haemochromatosis have been found to be homozygous for the same cysteine-to-tyrosine substitution at amino acid 282 in a novel major histocompatibility complex class I-like gene, called the *HLA-H* gene. The exact function of the protein that *HLA-H* codes for is unknown, but recent work suggests that the peptide is localized to a unique subcellular region in the crypts of the small intestine close to the sites of iron absorption.

Unfortunately, the incidence of *late primary hepatic carcinoma* is considerably elevated (20–30%) even if the patient is treated with adequate iron removal. Repeated venesection to bring ferritin down into the low normal range can restore cardiac and hepatic function, improve glucose tolerance and reduce skin pigmentation. The 5-year survival is 90%.

Basic science

Iron

A normal diet contains 5–15 mg of iron daily, mostly in red meat, liver and kidney, and of that about 1 mg is absorbed from the duodenum and proximal jejunum to compensate for losses from the skin, gastrointestinal and genitourinary tracts. Absorption of iron from the gut depends on the amount and bioavailability of iron and on the gut mucosa, which regulates iron absorption through unknown mechanisms. There are no specific physiological mechanisms for the excretion of iron.

Most of the body iron is locked up in the porphyrin complex of haemoglobin, with smaller quantities complexed to make myoglobin. Excess iron is stored as ferritin, in which a core of oxidized iron, Fe^{3+}, is deposited within an apoferritin protein envelope, and as haemosiderin, an aggregated and degraded form of ferritin. Iron is stored predominantly in the liver, spleen and bone marrow, and moved between compartments by the plasma protein transferrin.

There is a close correlation between circulating ferritin levels and total body iron. A low

Table 42.1 Iron content of some raw foods (mg per 100 g)

Food	mg per 100 g
Beef	1.9
Liver	11.4
White bread	1.7
Wholemeal bread	3.0
White flour	2.1
Red wine	0.8

ferritin level is diagnostic of iron deficiency anaemia. In haemochromatosis, there is deregulation of iron absorption from the gut, leading to progressive, massive iron absorption, very high ferritin levels (typically 900–6000 ng mL^{-1}; normal range, men = 15–400 ng mL^{-1}) and deposition of iron into the liver, pancreas, heart and pituitary gland with eventual tissue damage and functional insufficiency.

MCQs

1 A low ferritin level is diagnostic of iron deficiency.
2 Haemochromatosis is inherited as an autosomal recessive condition.
3 Hypogonadism is associated with haemochromatosis.
4 The pigmentation in haemochromatosis is due to the deposition of iron in the skin.
5 Free iron is removed from the circulation by binding to tissue haemosiderin and ferritin.

Case 43
A lifetime of diarrhoea

History

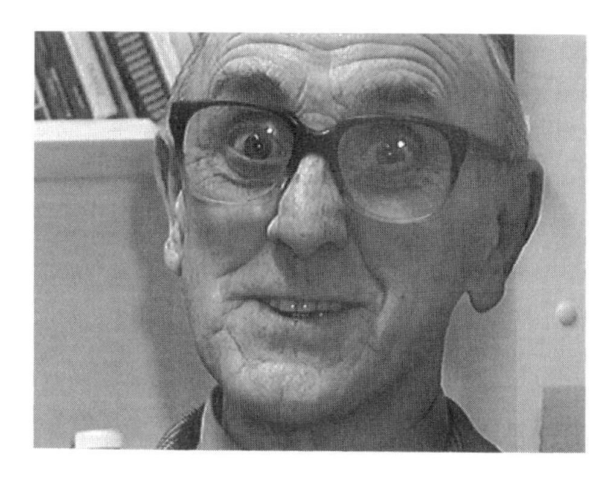

A 76-year-old retired fireman was seen in clinic with malabsorption. His history went back to an episode in childhood when he drank water from a stream and suffered from a severe attack of diarrhoea and vomiting 2 days later. From that time on, he had suffered from a **distended abdomen** (seen clearly in a picture taken with his brother at the age of 8 years), loose stools, urgency of bowel opening and difficulty flushing the stools away. The problem so affected his childhood that, after a number of accidents and close shaves, he was given special dispensation at school to visit the lavatory whenever he chose. After a 'B4' medical classification in the army and a posting to northern France in the Second World War, he had a successful career in the fire-fighting service. His symptoms continued as before and were not investigated until his sixth decade, when recurrent crops of severe aphthous mouth ulcers led to a referral to a dental hospital to determine whether sharp edges on his molars were causing the problem. A dental student noted that he had 'splits in the skin at the corners of his mouth' and suggested that he visit his doctor to exclude malabsorption. Blood tests revealed macrocytic anaemia and a series of investigations led to the diagnosis.

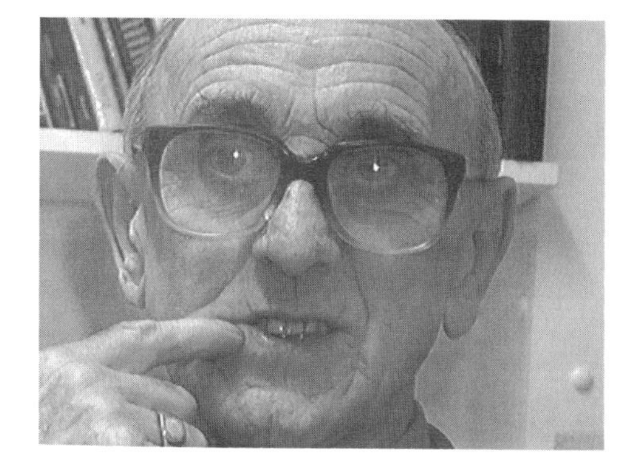

Notes

The patient had gluten-induced enteropathy (**coeliac disease**).

The history, physical findings (abdominal distension, **angular stomatitis** and steatorrhoea) and laboratory tests strongly suggested a diagnosis of malabsorption; gluten-induced enteropathy (coeliac disease or non-tropical sprue) was thought to be the most likely

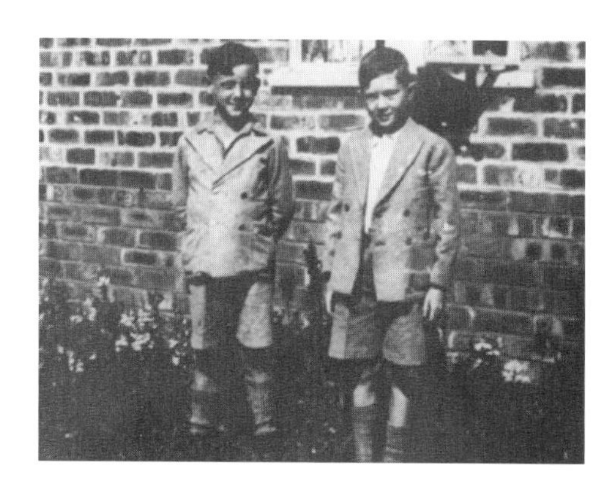

diagnosis. An oral gastroduodenoscopy was carried out and mucosal biopsies were taken which showed classical villus atrophy. With a strict gluten-free diet, his symptoms gradually abated over a period of several months, and the biochemical and haematological abnormalities began to return to normal.

Coeliac disease or gluten-induced enteropathy has a prevalence of around 0.1%, and is one of the most common causes of malabsorption in the UK population. The condition is strongly associated with the human leucocyte antigens HLA-DR3DQ2, HLA-DR5DR7 and HLA-DR4DQ8, with 10–20% of first degree relatives affected and concordance in monozygotic twins approaching 100%. Both coeliac disease and the related condition 'dermatitis herpetiformis' (characterized by an itchy, blistering rash affecting the back, buttocks, elbows and knees) improve with exclusion of gluten from the diet.

Whole wheat is separated by milling into an outer husk (bran), wheat germ (semolina) and flour (endosperm). The latter contains a number of proteins, including the non-toxic glutenins, globulins and albumins and the toxic gliadins which belong to the gluten group. Most of the toxicity of gliadins appears to be contained within the α subfraction, and most of the toxic effect is expended in the upper small intestine as the gluten is hydrolysed to a less toxic form during its distal progress. The result is various degrees of villous atrophy which can be asymptomatic or associated with, for example, a mild hypochromic, macrocytic anaemia with target cells (found particularly in liver disease, thalassaemia and sickle cell anaemia) and Howell–Jolly bodies (indicative of hyposplenism), unexplained osteoporosis or subfertility in adulthood, abdominal pain, anorexia and vomiting, weight loss, failure to thrive, diarrhoea and impaired growth in children. Other signs of malabsorption, such as hypoalbuminaemia and low folate levels, are also common, and, in severe diarrhoea, hypocalcaemia, hypomagnesaemia and sodium, potassium, zinc and copper deficiencies may also occur.

After 5 years of complete gluten exclusion from the diet (by avoiding wheat, barley, rye and possibly oats), the 10-fold increased risk of gastrointestinal tumours and 40-fold increased risk of intestinal lymphoma in coeliac disease return to normal.

Basic science

Malabsorption

Signs of nutritional deficiency in the face of adequate nutritional intake, particularly in the presence of abnormal stools, suggest malabsorption.

All of our nutritional requirements (possibly with the exception of vitamin D, which can be synthesized in the skin and is therefore not strictly a vitamin) are absorbed through the specialized mucosa of the gastrointestinal tract, after modification by a large number of digestive enzymes in the different micro-environments provided.

Carbohydrates. Principally polysaccharides (starches composed of polymers of glucose) and disaccharides (maltose, lactose (milk sugar) and sucrose (table sugar)) which are digested to monosaccharides (fructose (fruit sugar), glucose and galactose) and actively transported across the mucosa of the duodenum and ileum. Deficiency of the enzymes that break down disaccharides to monosaccharides, particularly lactase, is responsible for diarrhoea, bloating and flatulence after the ingestion of milk in many black races. The maximum rate of glucose absorption is $120\,g\,h^{-1}$ and depends on sodium in the lumen. Low sodium levels inhibit glucose absorption.

Proteins. Digestion begins in the stomach with gastric pepsins. These are inactivated when gastric juice enters the duodenum, but trypsin and chymotrypsin continue the process. A number of different transport systems are responsible for amino acid absorption, again facilitated by luminal sodium ions. Proteins are absorbed most rapidly in the duode-

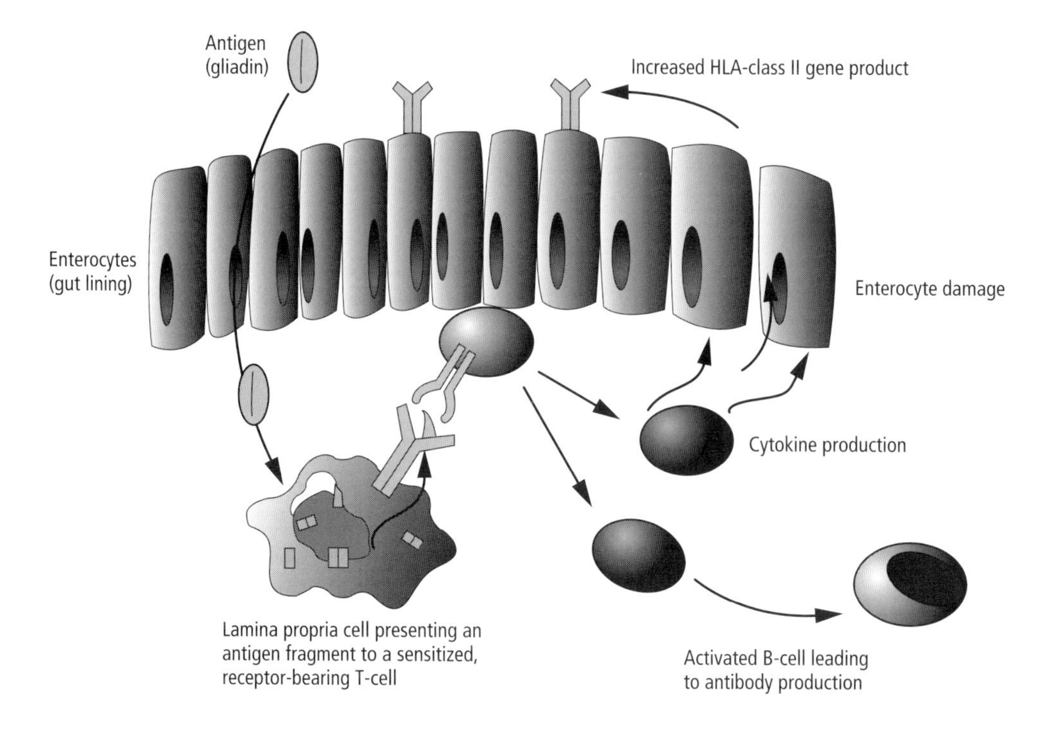

num and jejunum, and more slowly from the ileum. In infants, some whole proteins, such as immunoglobulins, are absorbed unchanged.

Lipids. Digestion begins in the duodenum. Pancreatic lipase is the most important enzyme, acting on fats emulsified by the action of bile salts, fatty acids and glycerides. Bile salts combine with fatty acids and monoglycerides to form micelles, which bring the lipids into close contact with the luminal surface, facilitating their absorption. The bile salts remain in the lumen and are absorbed in the terminal ileum. The absence of pancreatic lipase prevents the digestion of lipids even beginning, and results in fatty, bulky, clay-coloured, offensive stools often with oil droplets visible. Absorbed short chain fatty acids either enter the portal blood unchanged or are esterified together with long chain fatty acids in intestinal mucosal cells to triglycerides and formed into chylomicrons.

Vitamins. Absorption of fat-soluble vitamins is deficient if the absorption of fat is deficient, either because of pancreatic problems, lack of bile acids or mucosal abnormalities. Most vitamins are absorbed from the upper small intestine, with the exception of B_{12} which is absorbed from the terminal ileum.

Iron. Gastric acid is required to reduce ferric iron to ferrous iron, which is absorbed from the upper part of the small intestine.

Effects of nutritional deficiency

Calcium. Rickets in childhood and osteomalacia in adults. As calcium is present in many foods, vitamin D deficiency rather than calcium deficiency is usually responsible.

Potassium. Muscular weakness and lethargy.

Iron. Iron is required for the synthesis of haemoglobin, myoglobin and cytochromes that are essential for cellular respiration. Deficiency causes microcytic anaemia, weakness, angular stomatitis and koilonychia. Average iron loss is 1 mg per day (1.5 mg per day in women and up to 4 mg per day during the latter stages of pregnancy). A supplement of 100 mg per day is enough to provide a maximum haematopoietic response. An average daily diet contains 10–20 mg of iron, less than 10% of which is usually absorbed, mainly from the stomach and duodenum.

Thiamine. The deficiency disease is beriberi, characterized by tender, weak muscles, reduced reflexes, congestive cardiac failure and neuropathy. Wernicke's encephalopathy and Korsakoff's psychosis also occur.

Niacin or nicotinic acid. The deficiency disease is pellagra, characterized by diarrhoea, dermatitis and dementia.

Folic acid. Macrocytic anaemia and diarrhoea. Folate deficiency in pregnancy is also implicated in the failure of closure of the neural tube in early embryogenesis, with increased risk of anencephaly and spina bifida.

Vitamin B_{12}. Pernicious anaemia. Mild jaundice, diarrhoea, paraesthesia and subacute combined degeneration causing ataxia and mental changes. Liver, meat, eggs and milk are major dietary sources of this vitamin.

Vitamin C. Scurvy. Citrus fruits, green vegetables and potatoes contain large amounts of this water-soluble and heat-labile vitamin. In scurvy, there is impaired vascular integrity with petechiae, ecchymoses, painful subperiosteal haemorrhages and bleeding gums with tooth loss. The hairs on the lower abdomen can become tightly curled owing to folliculitis.

Vitamin D. Vital to facilitate the absorption of calcium and phosphate from the gut. Absence of vitamin D causes calcium deficiency, leading to rickets in childhood, osteomalacia in adulthood and neuromuscular excitability as ionized calcium levels fall.

Vitamin K. Vital for the synthesis of clotting factors II, VII, IX and X. The absence of vitamin K, or the excessive use of effective vitamin K antagonists (such as warfarin), causes increased prothrombin time and predisposition to haemorrhage.

Copper. Necessary for haemoglobin and cytochrome synthesis. Packed red cells contain about 100 μg copper per 100 mL. The plasma copper-carrying protein is ceruloplasmin. Most excretion of copper is in the stools. Nutritional deficiency has not been demonstrated in humans.

Iodine. Iodine deficiency causes hypothyroidism and endemic goitre. Cretinism results if the deficiency is congenital.

Cobalt. Affects blood formation. Used by microbes to synthesize B_{12}.

Zinc. Wound healing. Insulin contains zinc.

MCQs

1 A normal serum ferritin level excludes iron deficiency.
2 The prevalence of gluten-induced enteropathy in the general population is 1 : 1000.
3 Dermatitis herpetiformis, like coeliac disease, improves with a gluten-free diet.
4 In gluten-induced enteropathy, the ileum is as severely affected as the duodenum.
5 Gluten-induced enteropathy is associated with an increased risk of gastrointestinal tumours.

Case 44
Bloody diarrhoea and abdominal pains

History

A 30-year-old doorman, barman and labourer was admitted to hospital with a 6-week history of intermittent, but severe, abdominal pains associated with the passage of **bloody diarrhoea** up to 17 times daily. He had previously been completely well apart from mild, lower backache and some soreness of his eyes, and was very surprised when mild rectal discomfort ('like itching') was followed by the passage of large amounts of fresh, red blood per rectum. The pain would come on with very little warning and, unless he was able to immediately find a lavatory, the blood would stream down his legs accompanied sometimes by small amounts of loose stools and mucus. He denied a history of jaundice or gastroenteritis and, although he had not noticed a change in his appetite, had lost 14 lb in weight over the previous few weeks.

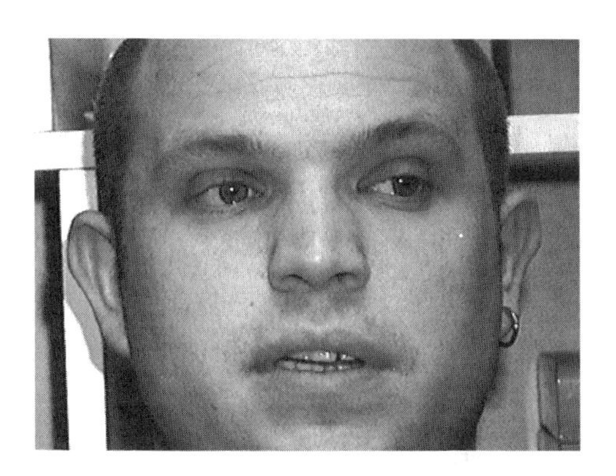

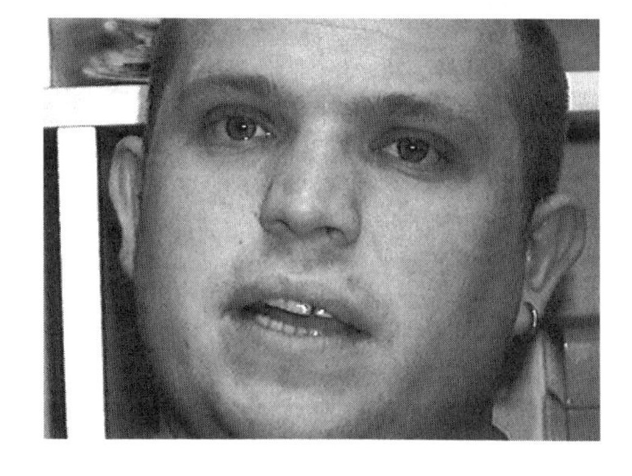

Notes

The patient had developed extensive ulcerative colitis.

Ulcerative colitis is a chronic, relapsing inflammatory disease of unknown aetiology that affects the large bowel. It starts at the rectum and extends proximally to involve part or all of the large intestine. There may be a history of atopy (asthma, eczema or hay fever) or autoimmune disease in affected patients. Ten per cent of patients have a first degree relative with the condition.

During relapses of the condition and, depending on the length of the segment of colon involved, there is *diarrhoea*, sometimes accompanied by the passage of *mucus* and *blood per rectum*, and systemic upset with malaise, fever, weight loss and abdominal pain. Complications include:

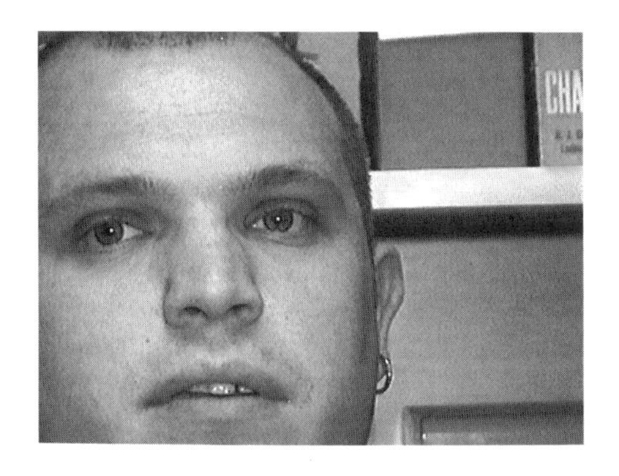

- toxic megacolon,
- perforation,
- haemorrhage,
- the development of colonic carcinoma (10–15% of patients with extensive disease after 20 years).

Extraintestinal complications include sacroiliitis and spondylitis, erythema nodosum and pyoderma gangrenosum, uveitis and episcleritis, sclerosing cholangitis, cholangiocarcinoma and a tendency to venous and arterial thrombosis.

Basic science

Differential diagnosis of bloody diarrhoea

- Diverticulitis.
- Colorectal cancer.
- Inflammatory bowel disease:
  - Ulcerative colitis.
  - Crohn's disease.
- Infective colitis:
  - *Campylobacter*, *Shigella*, *Salmonella*, *Clostridium difficile*, *Yersinia* and *E. coli*. Amoebiasis, schistosomiasis (*Schistosoma mansoni*), cytomegalovirus and herpes infections also cause bloody diarrhoea.
- Irradiation.
- Ischaemia.
- Behçet's disease.

Crohn's disease

Ulcerative colitis and Crohn's disease affect 0.1% of the population and may represent opposite poles of the same spectrum of genetically and environmentally induced disease. A number of factors clearly distinguish their natural histories and responses to treatment, including the observation that 66% of patients with Crohn's disease smoke, whereas ulcerative colitis occurs almost exclusively in nonsmokers. Crohn's disease can affect any part of the gastrointestinal tract, the most frequently involved site being the ileocaecal region, and, unlike ulcerative colitis, Crohn's disease responds to dietary therapy and metronidazole. Unlike Crohn's disease, inflammation of the bowel is confined to the colon in ulcerative colitis and surgery is curative. Both ulcerative colitis and Crohn's disease are associated with a number of extraintestinal complications, including erythema nodosum, reactive arthritis, ankylosing spondylitis and (extremely rarely) episcleritis. With the exception of ankylosing spondylitis, most of these problems resolve following successful treatment of the gastrointestinal disease with surgery, corticosteroids and dietary manipulation. Approximately one-half of the patients with Crohn's disease remain symptom free for 5 years after surgical resection of a segment of strictured bowel, and the use of 5-aminosalicylates and the cessation of smoking can further modestly reduce the risk of relapse.

Diarrhoea—colon function

The muscle of the colon is arranged circumferentially and in several longitudinal bands, which together are responsible for its sacculated appearance. Rhythmic segmentation and slow non-propulsive peristalsis mix the ingress of approximately 1 L of small bowel content daily. Propulsive peristalsis, a coordinated peristaltic rush that sweeps distally from the caecum, occurs two or three times daily, sometimes triggered by a meal (gastrocolic reflex). The resulting distension of the rectal walls results in a call to stool. In general, food residue remains in the colon for between 12 h and 3 days, while water, salts and water-soluble vitamins are absorbed. The brown colour of normal faeces is the result of stercobilin, the oxidation product of stercobilinogen in bile. In the absence of bile, stools are greyish-white. The characteristic odour is produced by the fermentation and putrefaction of carbohydrates and proteins (respectively) by aerobic and anaerobic bacteria that normally colonize the large bowel.

Diarrhoea is the production of abnormally frequent or loose stools for an individual.

Definitions based on volume may be less useful than definitions based on mechanism. In secretory diarrhoea, the absorption of electrolytes by the colonic mucosa and the loss of electrolytes through the mucosa are increased. Examples are cholera and bile salt-induced enteropathy in patients in whom the terminal ileum is unable to absorb irritant bile salts before their passage through the ileocaecal valve. Exudative diarrhoea is characteristic of ulcerative colitis and infections with *Shigella* and *Entamoeba histolytica*. Decreased absorption occurs in osmotic diarrhoea, such as in lactase deficiency and in the use of magnesium-containing cathartics, in anatomic problems that reduce absorptive surface area, such as colonic resection, and in motility disorders, such as irritable bowel syndrome and hyperthyroidism.

MCQs

1 Ulcerative colitis may be localized to the proximal large bowel.
2 Ulcerative colitis has a significant hereditary component.
3 Under normal circumstances, food residue remains within the colon for 4–12 h.
4 Bile salts are usually absorbed in the caecum and ascending colon.
5 Irritable bowel syndrome is a cause of exudative diarrhoea.

Case 45
Forgetfulness and morning sickness

History

A 46-year-old unemployed man was admitted to hospital with a history of nausea on waking in the morning and increasingly bad short-term memory. Over the previous 6 months, he had noticed the occasional passage of fresh, red blood when opening his bowels, but the stools themselves looked normal (rather than black). He claimed that his former wife had given him hepatitis B, but that he had not been jaundiced in the past except during an episode which he took to be influenza. At one time his abdomen had increased markedly in size. The symptom that interfered most with his lifestyle was that he found it impossible to concentrate at the best of times and, when he felt particularly unwell, his short-term memory seemed almost non-existent.

On examination, he was orientated and cooperative. There were some large spider naevi on his chest and head, bruising on his legs and an infected meibomian cyst. Abdominal examination revealed minimal ascites and a 2-cm liver edge. The tip of his spleen was also palpable. He did not have Dupuytren's contracture, gynaecomastia or testicular atrophy.

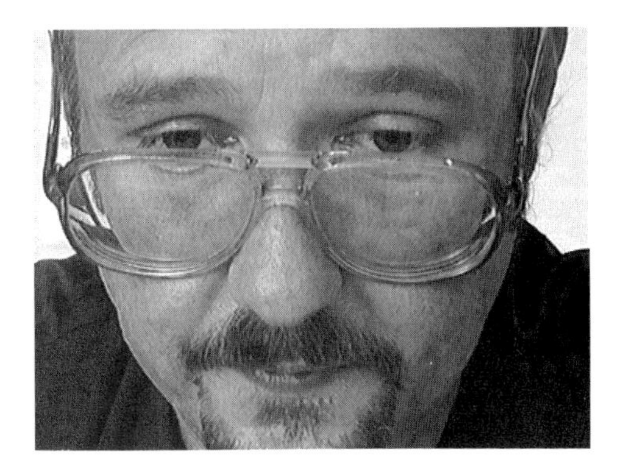

Notes

The patient had hepatic cirrhosis secondary to excessive alcohol ingestion. Serological tests for hepatitis B and C serology were negative.

He had previously been a bar owner, a very high risk profession for alcoholism, and showed many of the signs of chronic liver disease. Typical features are:

- jaundice,
- cachexia,
- parotid gland enlargement,
- Dupuytren's contracture,
- gynaecomastia,
- testicular atrophy, and
- diminished secondary sexual hair.

There may be bruising and purpura, palmar erythema and spider naevi above the umbilicus. Finger clubbing is relatively unusual, and scratch marks suggest chronic cholestasis, typical of biliary cirrhosis. A flapping tremor (asterixis) and confusion suggest hepatic encephalopathy. Ascites may be present on abdominal examination, and the presence of splenomegaly suggests portal hypertension or hepatitis. A palpable gallbladder suggests extrahepatic biliary obstruction (Courvoisier's sign, typical of carcinoma of the head of the pancreas), and tenderness over the gallbladder on palpation (Murphy's sign) suggests cholelithiasis particularly when complicated by cholecystitis. Defects in higher mental function, including short-term memory, are characteristic and form part of Korsakoff's psychosis.

Basic science

For *Alcohol* (Basic science), see Case 48 on p. 131. The other major cause of liver cirrhosis is infection with the hepatitis B virus.

Hepatitis B is a DNA virus that belongs to a group of so-called hepadnaviruses (short for hepatotrophic, DNA viruses). They all replicate within the liver, contain their own DNA polymerase and are associated with acute and chronic hepatitis and hepatocellular carcinoma. All body fluids are laden with viral particles. Mother to child **spread** is common, and infection through contact with semen and saliva is well described.

After a non-specific influenza-like prodrome, the patient often develops symptoms of cholestasis (dark urine and clay-coloured stools) followed 1–5 days later by jaundice. The liver is often enlarged and tender, reflecting hepatocellular necrosis with mononuclear cell infiltrate. In uncomplicated cases, complete clinical and biochemical recovery occurs within 4 months.

Hepatitis B surface antigen begins to appear in the plasma about 4 weeks after infection, rising to a peak at 3 months, followed by rising immunoglobulin M (IgM) antibody titres to core antigen (IgM Anti HBcAg) which appear at 6 weeks and reach high levels by 4–5 months.

Hepatitis C is an RNA virus responsible for 90% of cases of non-A, non-B hepatitis. It is a major cause of hepatic cirrhosis and hepatoma in many parts of the world. Only 10% of patients newly infected with hepatitis C become jaundiced, the development of chronic fatigue being a more typical feature of the infection. In 20–30% of infected individuals, complications such as cirrhosis develop over a period of 20–30 years although, in some patients, progression may be much quicker. Intravenous drug users exposed to contaminated blood through needle sharing are particularly at risk, as are patients who received large amounts of blood products before hepatitis C first became diagnosable by antibody tests in 1991. Interferon-α, the mainstay of treatment, induces normalization of alanine aminotransferase in fewer than 50% of patients, and the response is sustained in only 20%. Very few patients become virus free.

Table 45.1 The hepatitis viruses

Hepatitis virus	Transmission	Treatment
A	Enteral	Supportive
B	Parenteral Sexual contact Mother to child	Interferon Nucleoside analogues
C	Parenteral	Interferon
D	Parenteral with hepatitis B virus	Interferon Nucleoside analogues
E	Enteral	Supportive
G	Parenteral	None
Seronegative	Unknown	Supportive

MCQs

1 Transamination allows amino acids to enter the citric acid cycle.
2 Hepatitis C is the cause of 90% of cases of non-A, non-B viral hepatitis.
3 Hypoglycaemia is a feature of fulminant hepatic failure.
4 The memory defects of Korsakoff's syndrome recover with abstention from alcohol.
5 Treatment of hepatitis C with interferon-α renders 20% of patients virus free.

Case 46

Haematemesis and painful, weak muscles

History

A 46-year-old unemployed barman was admitted to casualty with a short history of haematemesis. He had been drinking his third pint of beer in a pub when he suddenly became nauseated and vomited violently. After the initial blood-free vomit, he subsequently vomited four cupfuls of fresh red blood, felt faint and 'collapsed' to the ground.

On examination, he was noted to have sores on his skin and **multiple bruises** over his legs and chest, and spider naevi on his chest and forehead. His blood pressure and pulse, which were taken immediately after his arrival in casualty, were 134/86 mmHg and 72 beats per minute, respectively. Fine nystagmus was evident on lateral gaze, and there appeared to be mild, diffuse muscular weakness, although this was difficult to confirm. During the examination he vomited 'coffee grounds' (changed blood). Examination of his abdomen, chest, genitals and rectum was normal.

His full blood count showed a haemoglobin level of 12.2 $g\,dL^{-1}$ (normal range = 11.5–15.5 $g\,dL^{-1}$) with a mean corpuscular volume (MCV) of 101 fL (83–96 fL) and platelet count of $311 \times 10^9\,L^{-1}$ ($(150–400) \times 10^9\,L^{-1}$). Subsequent results showed a blood urea level of 7 $mmol\,L^{-1}$ (3–7 $mmol\,L^{-1}$), alkaline phosphatase of 100 $U\,L^{-1}$ (20–120 $U\,L^{-1}$), aspartate aminotransferase of 30 $U\,L^{-1}$ (6–35 $U\,L^{-1}$) and γ-glutamyl transpeptidase (γ-GT) of 162 $U\,L^{-1}$ (6–32 $U\,L^{-1}$). An upper gastrointestinal endoscopy carried out within 12 h of admission was entirely normal. The patient remembered very little of the episode.

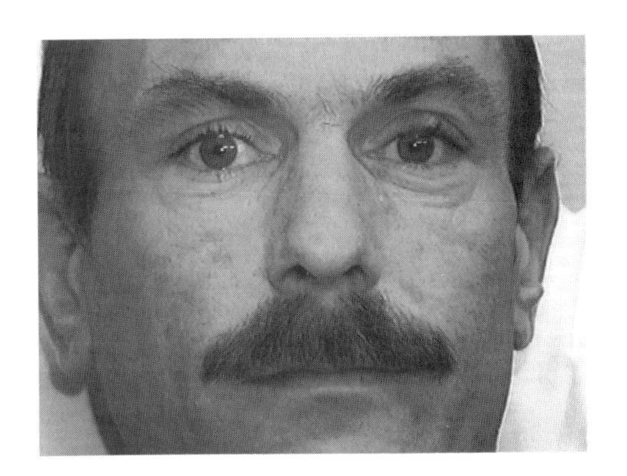

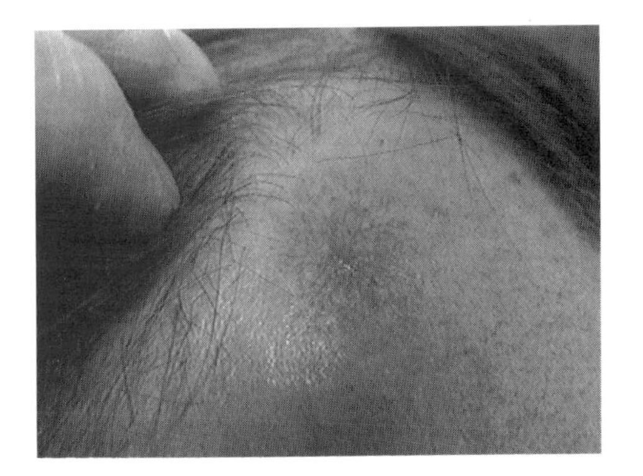

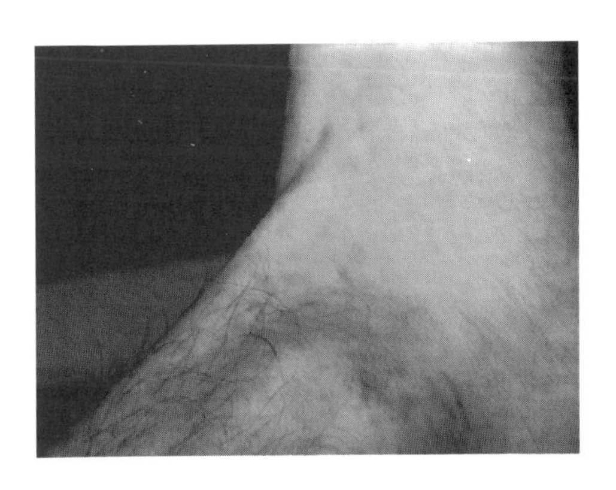

Notes

The patient had a Mallory–Weiss tear.

A Mallory–Weiss tear is a mucosal rather than a transmural tear that usually involves the gastric mucosa in the region of the cardia. It is caused by violent retching, characteristic of patients who ingest excessive amounts of alcohol. The characteristic history is of a violent, blood-free vomit followed, on subsequent vomiting, by frank haematemesis. The tear usually heals remarkably rapidly and, in most cases, no lesion is seen on subsequent endoscopy.

Haemodilution takes time to occur and, in this patient, shortly after a single, acute episode of blood loss, the haemoglobin reflected the state prior to haemorrhage. The 'collapse' that followed his haematemesis was the result of parasympathetic stimulation (i.e. a vasovagal episode or faint) that commonly accompanies haematemesis, rather than hypovolaemic shock. The raised MCV is characteristic of heavy, prolonged alcohol ingestion, as is the elevated γ-GT. Nutritional deficiency is common in alcoholics, and acute neurological problems related to thiamine deficiency, although rare, are anticipated in their treatment.

Basic science

Thiamine deficiency

In the mitochondria of aerobic cells, two-carbon residues produced by the breakdown of carbohydrates, fatty acids and amino acids are oxidized to form acetyl-coenzyme A (acetyl-CoA) and metabolized to produce carbon dioxide, water and energy in the citric acid (Krebs') cycle and its accompanying respiratory chain. In this self-regenerating chain of reactions, each two-carbon acetyl-CoA molecule entering is condensed with four-carbon oxaloacetate to produce citrate. Two carbon dioxide molecules are cleaved from citrate within the cycle to regenerate four-carbon oxaloacetate ready to react with the next molecule of acetyl-CoA entering. The pairs of hydrogen atoms split off power oxidative phosphorylation, producing adenosine triphosphate (ATP) from adenosine diphosphate (ADP) and Pi.

Without thiamine (vitamin B_1), pyruvate cannot be oxidized to acetyl-CoA, glucose cannot be utilized aerobically and pyruvic and lactic acids accumulate—a state exacerbated by a high carbohydrate diet (such as one consisting mostly of beer). As the dietary intake of thiamine is marginal and little of the water-soluble vitamin is stored in the body, alcoholics are prone to develop classical thiamine deficiency.

The consequences are impairment of neuronal and muscular function, resulting in *neuropathy*, *encephalopathy* and *cardiomyopathy*. Accumulation of lactic and pyruvic acids causes vasodilatation which, added to impaired glucose utilization, produces high output cardiac failure.

Wernicke's encephalopathy presents as ophthalmoplegia and impaired consciousness caused by foci of congestion and petechial haemorrhages in the upper midbrain, hypothalamus, walls of the third ventricle and mammillary bodies. *Korsakoff's psychosis*, disorientation, severe short-term memory impairment and delusions often accompany Wernicke's encephalopathy.

Thiamine deficiency is the cause of *beriberi* (Singhalese for 'weakness'). In dry beriberi, produced by thiamine deficiency in the absence of carbohydrate, there is severe muscle wasting and degeneration and demyelination of nerves. The presence of carbohydrate leads to the accumulation of pyruvic and lactic acids (because of a lack of pyruvate decarboxylase), profound peripheral vasodilatation, oedema and high output cardiac failure with congestive cardiomyopathy, which further exacerbates oedema (so-called wet beriberi).

MCQs

1 Thiamine is a cofactor required for the carboxylic acid (Krebs') cycle.
2 Differences in carbohydrate intake

affect the manifestation of thiamine deficiency.

3 Wernicke's encephalopathy, Korsakoff's psychosis and pellagra are all manifestations of thiamine deficiency.

4 A Mallory–Weiss tear is a transmural tear of the junction of the stomach and lower oesophagus.

5 Diplopia is a typical feature of Wernicke's encephalopathy.

Case 47
Heartburn and a lifetime of antacids

History

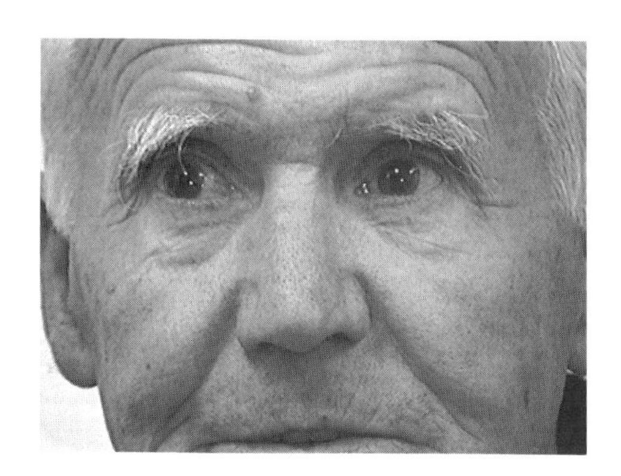

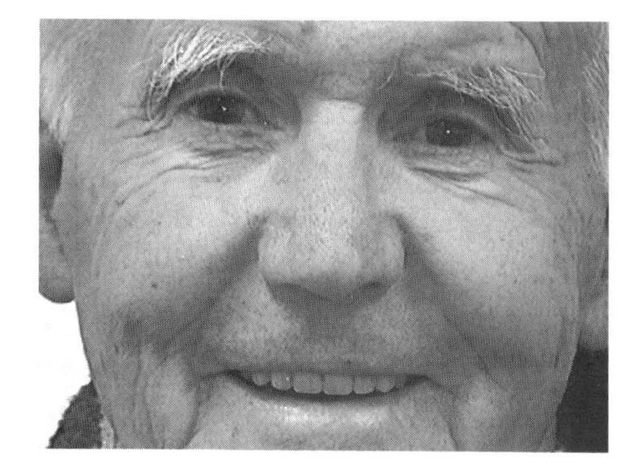

A 75-year-old retired factory worker was admitted to hospital with a history of developing nausea and vomiting after eating a salad. He vomited a number of times and, although not particularly disturbed by the episode itself, noted that the vomit was black. He reported this to his doctor who ignored his protests that the discoloration was probably due to iron tablets, and referred him directly to casualty. The patient had suffered throughout his adult life from the reflux of burning gastric acid which would occur at any time, but particularly after eating or on bending down. This had been controlled by copious ingestion of antacids from when he first joined the army at the age of 18 years. He had put up with the symptoms for many years, and denied any episodes of haematemesis or melaena. On one occasion, 16 years previously, he had visited his doctor for a prescription for antacids and had been given a blood test which showed that he had mild iron deficiency anaemia. An endoscopy showed 'four small **gastric ulcers**' and, from that time on, he had taken iron tablets as well as antacids. For the last two decades, he had been slightly less troubled by gastric acid reflux and, on proton pump inhibitors prescribed by his doctor, had become almost symptom free.

Notes

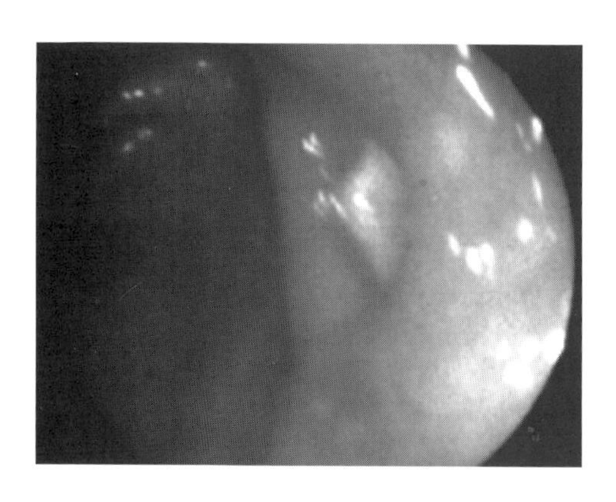

The patient had gastro-oesophageal reflux disease complicated by bleeding from a duodenal ulcer.

Symptoms of gastro-oesophageal reflux disease affect 7–10% of the adult population on a daily basis. The pathology ranges from severe inflammation and ulceration of the lower oesophagus, which can lead to stricture formation, through to asymptomatic reflux without mucosal damage which is 5–10 times more common. Symptomatically, patients can complain of burning, retrosternal discomfort (heartburn), the sensation of reflux into the oesophagus, pain on swallowing, particularly hot fluids, and dysphagia due to peptic stricture. In addition to dysphagia, sinister features include an age of onset of over 45 years, weight loss, haematemesis and melaena, and vomiting. Drugs such as non-steroidal anti-inflammatories, potassium chloride and some bisphosphonates can also exacerbate oesophagitis.

Basic science

Helicobacter pylori

Helicobacter pylori is a curved, Gram-negative rod bacterium first identified in 1982. By having 4–6 flagella at one end to allow for motility within the gastric mucous layer and by expressing a proton pump to control its intracellular pH and a urease to facilitate the breakdown of urea into ammonia (forming alkaline ammonium hydroxide in solution), it is well adapted to live in the extremely harsh environment of the stomach. The route of initial colonization is unclear, but the event is associated with temporary achlorhydria. Strains producing vacuolating toxin (vacA) are highly correlated with chronic gastritis and with gastric ulcers, gastric cancer and lymphoma. Over 90% of duodenal ulcers are associated with *H. pylori* infection, and eradication of the organism is associated with a cure of the disease in most patients. Remarkably, lymphoma regression also occurs in a high proportion of patients after *H. pylori* eradication. The diagnosis is made by identifying urease action in biopsy specimens or ^{13}C- or ^{14}C-tagged carbon dioxide in the breath after ingestion of a bolus of ^{14}C urea.

Mechanism of duodenal ulcer formation

The gastric antrum contains 'G' cells, which produce gastrin in response to stimulation by food, and 'D' cells, which secrete somatostatin in response to gastric acid and complete the feedback loop by inhibiting gastrin production. *H. pylori* infection increases gastrin production and reduces somatostatin production. The increased acid load passes into the duodenum, producing metaplastic change to a pseudogastric mucosal conformation, which is, in turn, colonized by *H. pylori*, leading to duodenitis and ulceration.

MCQs

1 Infection with *H. pylori* produces temporary achlorhydria.
2 *H. pylori* can be identified indirectly by looking for evidence of specific enzyme activity.
3 *H. pylori* is a curved, Gram-positive rod bacterium.
4 Over 90% of duodenal ulcers are associated with *H. pylori* infection.
5 *H. pylori* is associated with gastric carcinoma and lymphoma formation.

Case 48

Jaundice and disorientation

History

A 42-year-old bar owner was admitted to hospital with a 4-day history of increasing jaundice and a 24-h history of drowsiness and disorientation. He had served a 5-year term in the armed forces before leaving to run a bar, and, for more than 25 years, had consumed between 3 and 8 pints of beer per day. For the 2 years before the current episode, he had been admitted to hospital increasingly frequently, complaining of episodes of jaundice and abdominal distension. His brother who lived some distance away but visited regularly, noted that, on this occasion, the patient had developed anorexia, diarrhoea and rapidly worsening disorientation and jaundice.

On examination, he was markedly jaundiced, had multiple spider naevi and a moderate amount of ascites. He was apyrexial, but disorientated in place and person, and was unable to even give an approximation of his age on direct questioning without reference to his brother who was by the bedside. A flapping tremor of his outstretched hands was clearly visible.

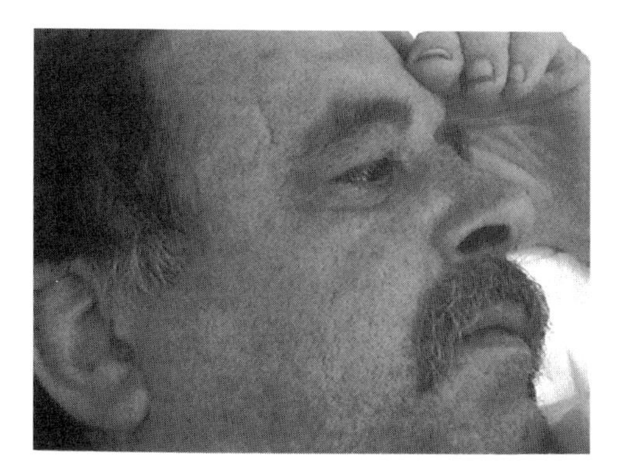

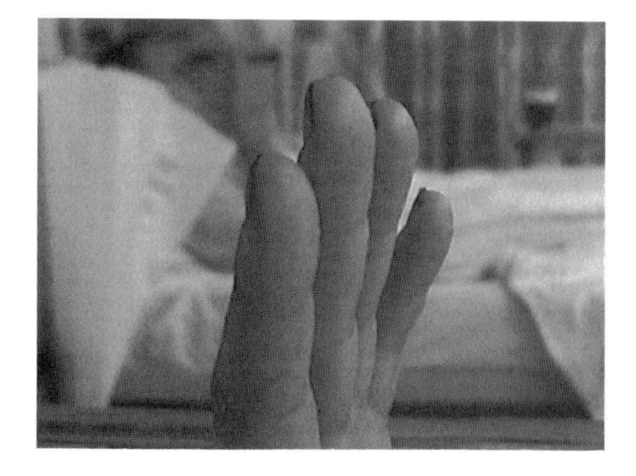

Notes

The patient had developed **hepatic encephalopathy** as a complication of alcohol-induced cirrhosis.

Hepatic encephalopathy is a complex neuropsychiatric syndrome arising from the passage of gut-derived neurotoxins through or around a diseased liver into the systemic circulation and across a dysfunctional blood–brain barrier. It is associated with reduced cerebral blood flow and decreased cerebral consumption of glucose and oxygen. Specific pathogenic factors remain unknown, but ammonia, mercaptans from the metabolism of methionine by the gut, short chain fatty acids, phenol and γ-aminobutyric acid (GABA) have all been implicated.

The principal clinical effects are reduced conscious level and behavioural and personality changes, with fluctuating neurological signs and a flapping tremor. Daytime somnolence, loss of self-care and disturbances of awareness, thinking and memory, leading to confusion and eventual coma, are also characteristic. Asterixis (liver flap) is produced by repeated, non-rhythmic, transient loss of voluntarily sustained position control.

Encephalopathy is typically exacerbated by gastrointestinal bleeding, increased dietary protein intake, electrolyte disturbance (e.g. hypokalaemia, vomiting or the use of diuretics), surgical procedures such as paracentesis or infections (including superimposed hepatitis). The use of central nervous system suppressants, such as anaesthetics and sedatives, can worsen encephalopathy, as can hypoxia and biliary obstruction.

The following grades are recognized:

- *Grade 0*. No abnormality detected.
- *Grade I*. Euphoria or depression, mild confusion, slurred speech, sleep disturbance. Trivial lack of awareness, shortened attention span.
- *Grade II*. Lethargy, moderate confusion and liver flap. Disorientation in time and place, inappropriate behaviour.
- *Grade III*. Marked confusion, incoherent speech, sleeping but rousable. Liver flap. Gross disorientation.
- *Grade IV*. Coma. Mental state cannot be tested.

Basic science

Alcohol

Alcohol is absorbed principally from the proximal small intestine. The rate of absorption is increased by rapid gastric emptying, the absence of food, dilution to 20% by volume and carbonation. Between 2% (at low concentration) and 10% (at high concentration) of alcohol is excreted directly through the lungs. The majority is metabolized to acetaldehyde by the liver at the rate of about 1 unit per hour (10g). This rate can be increased by 30% with repeated exposure over a 1–2-week period.

Alcoholism

In the UK, 20% of the adult population consume 80% of the alcohol, 3% consume 30% and 300000 people are alcohol dependent. Between 8 and 10% of deaths in the 16- to 74-year-old age group are alcohol related, and 15–30% of men admitted to hospital have a significant alcohol problem (8–15% of women). The risk of a road traffic accident at the UK legal limit (80 mg L^{-1}) is 10 times normal, and suicide is 20 times more common in the alcoholic population.

Central effects of alcohol

At low concentrations, alcohol promotes the central action of GABA, leading to sedation and ataxia. The pleasurable effects are thought to be related to the release of amine neurotransmitters, such as dopamine, and endogenous opioids, such as endorphins. At higher concentrations, alcohol stimulates 5-HT_3 receptors, contributing to nausea and vomiting and, by blocking excitatory transmission through glutamate receptors, further deepening sedation and amnesia. The number of glutamate receptors is upregulated by continued alcohol use and, on withdrawal, their overactivity contributes to tremors, seizures and neuronal death, which leads eventually to alcoholic dementia.

MCQs

1 Hepatic encephalopathy can be reversible or chronic and progressive.
2 Hepatic dysfunction and/or portal blood shunting are prerequisites for encephalopathy.
3 Alkalosis tends to exacerbate hepatic encephalopathy.
4 The rate of alcohol metabolism increases as plasma levels rise.
5 Carbonation of drinks accelerates the absorption of alcohol.

Case 49
Painless, progressive jaundice

History

A 78-year-old retired farmer presented with a 2-week history of progressive, painless jaundice. He had previously been perfectly well and denied any physical symptoms, except that he had noticed that over the previous 2 weeks his urine had become dark and 'frothy' and his stools were slightly paler than before. He had experienced no contact with jaundiced people, had not travelled abroad and had not suffered any abdominal discomfort in the past. His appetite was unimpaired and he had not experienced any weight loss.

There were no abnormal findings on examination, other than marked jaundice and clay-coloured stools on rectal examination. In particular, abdominal examination was completely unremarkable and, apart from one or two scratch marks, there were no signs of chronic liver disease.

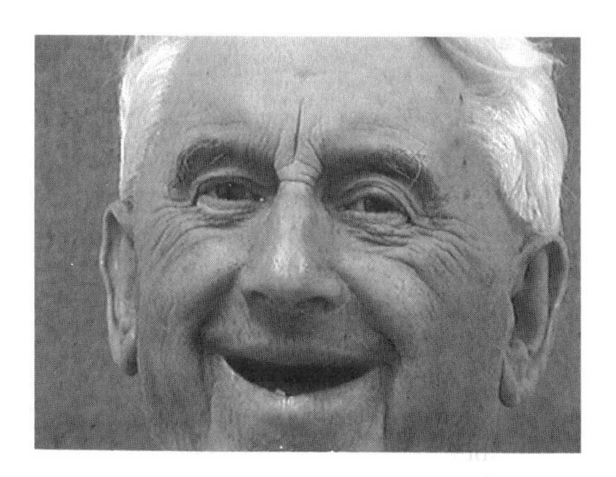

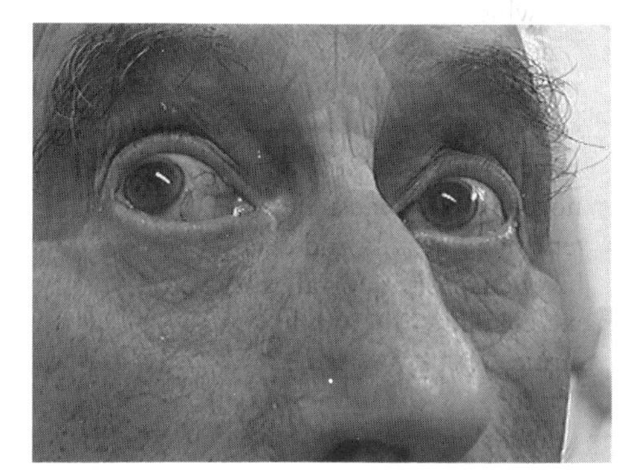

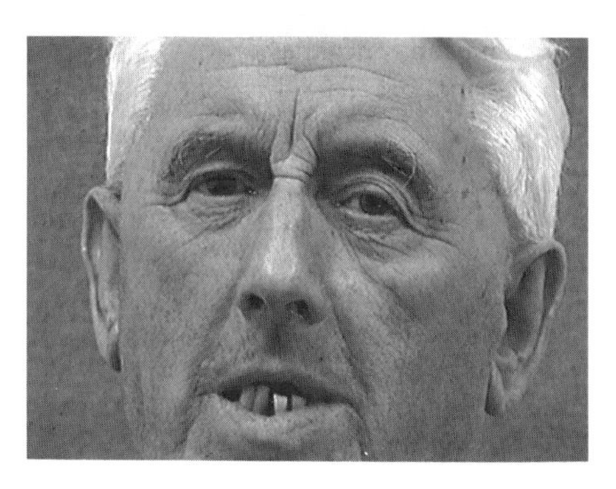

Notes

An ultrasound of the biliary tree and pancreas revealed a 4-cm tumour in the head of the pancreas with multiple, small hepatic metastases.

Pancreatic cancer is the fifth leading cause of cancer death in the UK. The incidence increases with age and the prognosis is very poor, with a negligible 5-year survival rate.

Classical presentation, as in the above patient, is with:
- painless obstructive jaundice,
- weight loss,
- upper abdominal pain, and
- a palpable gallbladder (Courvoisier's sign), in some cases.

In 65% of cases, the tumour arises from the head of the pancreas, and obstruction of the common bile duct, with jaundice, occurs early. In the 35% of tumours that arise in the body or tail of the pancreas, jaundice is a late sign and is more likely to result from extensive metastatic deposits than from common bile duct obstruction.

Basic science

Jaundice is often classified on the basis of the **pathogenic mechanism**—haemolytic, hepatocellular or obstructive. More than one mechanism may be involved, but one will often predominate.

Jaundice is yellow pigmentation of the skin and sclera by bilirubin. Bilirubin is the product of haemoglobin, 80% of which is derived from senescent red cells. The remaining 20% of bilirubin is derived from the direct destruction of maturing red cells in bone marrow and the turnover of haem and haem products in the liver. Haemoglobin is converted into haem, which is converted to biliverdin and then to bilirubin. Bilirubin is taken up by the liver, where glucuronyl transferase conjugates it to bilirubin monoglucuronide then diglucuronide, which is subsequently excreted into bile (an energy-dependent and rate-limiting step) and released into the duodenum. Conjugated bilirubin in the intestinal lumen is either excreted unchanged or metabolized to urobilinogen through the action of bacteria in the lower small intestine and colon, and partially reabsorbed into the portal circulation. Some is re-excreted into bile and the rest is excreted in the urine. Thus the presence of bilirubin products in the urine suggests that the hyperbilirubinaemia is conjugated.

Predominantly unconjugated hyperbilirubinaemia	
Overproduction	Haemolysis Ineffective erythropoiesis
Decreased hepatic uptake	Drugs Sepsis Starvation
Decreased hepatic conjugation	Gilbert's syndrome Crigler–Najjar Neonatal jaundice Drug induced Hepatitis Cirrhosis Sepsis

Predominantly conjugated hyperbilirubinaemia	
Decreased hepatic excretion into bile, either familial or acquired	Dubin–Johnson syndrome Rotor syndrome Cholestatic jaundice of pregnancy Viral or drug-induced hepatitis Drug induced, i.e. sex steroids Sepsis
Extrahepatic biliary obstruction	Gallstones Strictures Obstructing tumours

MCQs

1 Porphyrins are breakdown products of haemoglobin.
2 Jaundice associated with pale stools and dark urine is usually due to haemolysis.
3 Gut enzymes metabolize conjugated bilirubin in the intestinal lumen to urobilinogen.
4 Some bilirubin is derived directly from bone marrow activity.
5 Raised urinary bilirubin products are indicative of conjugated hyperbilirubinaemia.

Case 50
The hypnotherapy that didn't work

History

A 38-year-old mortgage administrator, who admitted to being a 'tense' person, was seen in the outpatient department with a 3-year history of intermittent loose stools, abdominal bloating, unproductive calls to stool and a feeling of incomplete emptying of the rectum after opening his bowels. He also complained of the occasional passage of fresh red blood after straining to open his bowels and of shooting abdominal pains, 'wind' and constipation. On the advice of a clinical ecologist who diagnosed allergies to alcohol, wheat, yeast and dairy products, he adopted a strict 'allergen-free diet' which had no effect on his symptoms, but made him lose 21 lb in body weight over a period of several months. He had also tried hypnotherapy, but could not afford to continue with the treatments or continue with the vitamin supplements that had been recommended. His past medical history consisted of a predisposition to headaches which had been diagnosed as migraine, and mild psoriasis which appeared in guttate form when he was 18 years of age. The occasional relapses of this condition also made him stressed. Examination was entirely normal.

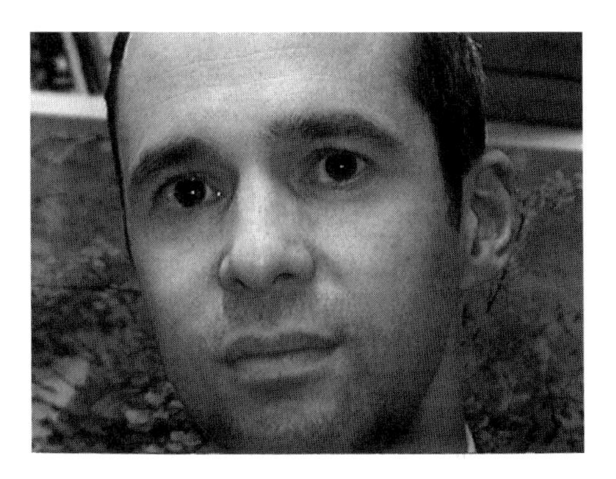

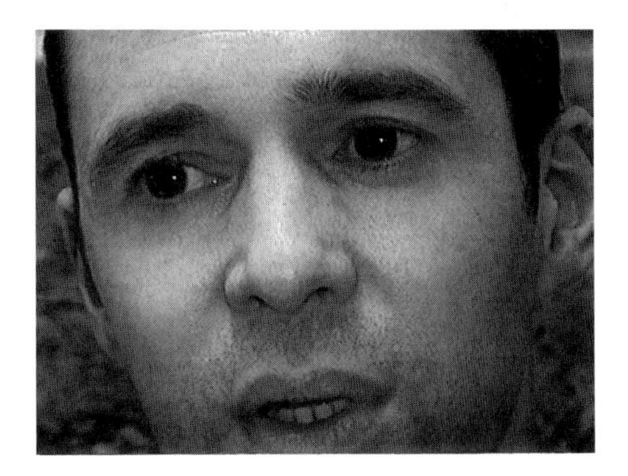

Notes

The patient had irritable bowel syndrome.

Irritable bowel disease is a very common syndrome characterized by a group of abdominal and defaecatory symptoms that occur in normal people, but cluster together more than by chance in patients with the condition. *Typical features* are:

- abdominal pain that decreases after defaecation (suggesting pain derived from the lower intestine),
- increased frequency and looseness of stools,
- abdominal pains,
- bloating and distension of the abdomen,
- a rectal feeling of incomplete emptying, and
- urgency and frequent calls to stool with intermittent constipation.

Importantly, the stools that are passed are usually normal and, if diarrhoea does occur, it is episodic rather than continuous. At least 13% of women and 5% of men have three or more of these symptoms which are thought to result from visceral hypersensitivity. Irritable bowel disease is a neurogastroenterological problem rather than a motility disorder. Patients who suffer from it are often polysymptomatic, and may be referred to gynaecologists with 'pelvic pain', to urologists with an irritable bladder, to neurologists with migraines and tension headaches and to general physicians with fatigue. Irritable bowel disease is not associated with constant abdominal pain or distension, constant diarrhoea, weight loss or the passage of blood with stool.

Basic science

Psychosomatic diseases, **personality disorders**, neuroses such as anxiety and depression and nervousness are common conditions encountered in general medical practice. Hypochondriacal neuroses, in which the patient is excessively preoccupied with bodily functions and physical symptoms such as bowel and urinary function, tinnitus, headaches, backache, potency and so on, are complicated by the physician's fear of missing an important underlying physical problem. Typical personality disorders that present with psychosomatic disease are the obsessive–compulsive personality, in which excessive inhibitions and failure to relax are complicated by tension in relationships and social isolation, the inadequate personality, in which a patient with no physical or intellectual problem is nevertheless unable to meet the demands of ordinary life, and the asthenic or neurasthenic personality, characterized by chronic weakness, exhaustion and fatiguability with poor response to stress.

Personality disorders, ranging from fearful, anxious or odd patients to the flamboyant or eccentric, occur in over 10% of urban adults, in 50% of psychiatric inpatients and in 60% of patients who present with parasuicide. Borderline personality disorder does not respond well to psychotherapy.

MCQs

1 Continuous diarrhoea is a typical symptom of irritable bowel syndrome.
2 Weight loss makes the diagnosis of irritable bowel syndrome unlikely.
3 Parasuicide is a poor predictor of personality disorder.
4 A feeling of incomplete emptying of the rectum after defaecation suggests ulcerative proctitis.
5 Symptoms associated with irritable bowel syndrome are common in the general population.

MCQ answers

Case 1

1 **False** The most common age of onset is between 24 and 32 years.
2 **True** These vitamin deficiencies are particularly associated with mental changes. Depression is characteristic.
3 **True** Unfortunately, this is indeed the case.
4 **True** Mental changes are often amongst the first symptoms of Cushing's disease, and hypothyroidism, particularly when it follows a period of thyrotoxicosis, is associated with depression.
5 **True** Dexamethasone fails to suppress endogenous glucocorticoids in 50% of cases, mimicking Cushing's syndrome.

Case 2

1 **False** Encephalopathy is not usually evident until 8–28 days after the onset of acute liver failure.
2 **False** The production of toxic intermediates continues unabated, but the reactive intermediates formed bind to *N*-acetylcysteine rather than to liver macromolecules.
3 **True** It is metabolism of the drug by the P_{450} enzyme systems in the liver that gives rise to its toxicity.
4 **True** Acetominophen poisoning has a number of effects, including pancreatitis, hypoglycaemia and cardiac damage.
5 **False** Unfortunately, there is little evidence to suggest that any intervention is useful.

Case 3

1 **False** ECG changes other than sinus tachycardia are unusual.
2 **False** Heparin does bind to antithrombin III, but it dramatically potentiates its activity.
3 **True** It antagonizes the hepatic production of the vitamin K-dependent clotting factors II, VII, IX and X.
4 **True** As it is a relatively invasive procedure, ventilation/perfusion scanning is more often used, although the sensitivity and specificity of this investigation are relatively poor.
5 **False** Most cases of pulmonary embolus occur without an obvious peripheral site of thrombosis.

Case 4

1 **True** This is one of the factors that accounts for the late presentation of patients with this disease.
2 **False** Stromal cell tumours, which account for 10% of ovarian tumours, are largely responsible for the hormone-secreting subtypes.
3 **False** Formation of the fallopian tubes, the uterus and the upper third of the vagina from the Müllerian ducts is entirely independent of ovarian development.
4 **True** The androgens are largely aromatized to oestrogens by granulosa cells that surround developing follicles.
5 **False** Vaginal lubrication is oestrogen dependent. Lack of oestrogens leads to dyspareunia.

Case 5

1 **False** In 50%, the disease develops in association with a respiratory tract infection over several days and, in 20%

of these, the time course is even longer.

2 **False** Neck stiffness, a cardinal sign of meningitis, is caused by muscle spasm.

3 **False** Pneumococcus and meningococcus are responsible for the majority of cases in adults. In children, *Haemophilus* is responsible for 50% of cases (2% in adults).

4 **False** Inflammation extends throughout the pia-arachnoid which surrounds the spinal cord, brain, cerebral ventricles, choroid plexus and cranial nerves.

5 **True** Encephalitis is a serious threat.

Case 6

1 **True** More than 10% of patients with peanut allergy have had to be admitted to hospital at some time with symptoms such as abdominal pain and collapse.

2 **True** Although environmental factors are important, 7% of siblings of patients with peanut allergy are also allergic to peanuts.

3 **False** There is little relationship between the test and clinical severity. As little as 100 μg of peanut protein can elicit a response.

4 **True** They are mediated by immunoglobulin E (IgE) antibodies bound to specific high affinity receptors on the surface of mast cells and basophils.

5 **False** Hypotension and cardiovascular collapse are more usual. It is more typical for ingested allergens to cause respiratory difficulty that progresses to asphyxia.

Case 7

1 **False** Bronchial breathing is heard in pulmonary fibrosis and consolidation. It is also characteristically heard over a small area at the top of pleural effusions.

2 **False** The anatomical dead space is usually about 150 mL—roughly equal to the body weight in pounds.

3 **False** By passing through poorly ventilated lung, blood in the pulmonary arteries reaches the pulmonary veins without being oxygenated. This can indeed cause arterial oxygen desaturation, but the shunt is right to left.

4 **False** Rapid, shallow breathing is adopted as the most pain-free and energy-efficient pattern of respiration.

5 **True** Production of surfactant is an extremely important function of type II pneumocytes.

Case 8

1 **False** Most patients recover uneventfully without long-term problems. About 20% of patients go on to chronic idiopathic thrombocytopenia and may require long-term treatment.

2 **False** They are usually either normal in number or increased.

3 **False** Spontaneous bleeding, even when the platelet count falls to $40 \times 10^9\,L^{-1}$, is uncommon. When the count reaches $20 \times 10^9\,L^{-1}$, spontaneous bleeding is common and, below $10 \times 10^9\,L^{-1}$, it is often severe.

4 **False** Iron deficiency is not associated with thrombocytopenia.

5 **False** It is regulated by the hormone thrombopoietin.

Case 9

1 **False** Neither is myeloma the result of a proliferation of B lymphocytes, strictly speaking, as such a proliferation would give rise to leukaemia. The cell involved is the terminally differentiated, antibody-producing form of B cell called a plasma cell.

2 **True** Anaemia and uraemia are poor prognostic signs in myelomatosis.

3 **False** Hypercalcaemia does cause constipation, but polyuria is more typical. Dehydration is a very characteristic feature of marked hypercalcaemia, and

rehydration is an important part of emergency treatment of the condition.

4 **True** And hy*PO*calcaemia is associated with a *PRO*longed Q–T interval (the interval from the beginning of the QRS complex to the beginning of the T wave). ECG signs are often mild and occur late in the condition.

5 **False** Although this tends to be true of breast cancer, in most other malignancies hypercalcaemia results from the production of parathyroid hormone-related peptide or other calcaemic factors.

Case 10

1 **True** Intermittent claudication is a good indicator of arterial disease elsewhere.

2 **False** It is one of the most effective and beneficial measures in peripheral vascular disease.

3 **False** Cartilage and epithelia receive nutrients from blood vessels in neighbouring tissues, and the cornea is entirely avascular.

4 **False** Fenestrated capillaries, which are found in the small intestine and endocrine glands, allow digested nutrients or hormones, respectively, to enter the bloodstream. The blood–brain barrier is characterized by continuous capillaries with endothelial cell perimeters bounded by tight junctions.

5 **False** Postcapillary venules are very permeable.

Case 11

1 **False** In complete heart block, the electrical dissociation between the atria and ventricles is complete.

2 **True** If the pacemaker is near the His bundle, it continues to be influenced by parasympathetic tone and the rate will increase to some extent with exercise, breathing and emotions.

3 **True** Stimulation of the carotid sinus, particularly in elderly patients, may indeed cause sinus arrest or such marked bradycardia that the patient may briefly lose consciousness.

4 **False** Vomiting is associated with an increase in vagal tone and bradycardia.

5 **True** When the idioventricular pacemaker moves from one part of the ventricle to another, temporary asystole may occur.

Case 12

1 **False** In these patients, the absolute risk of increased circulating low density lipoprotein (LDL) cholesterol is more strongly associated with cardiovascular disease than is smoking.

2 **False** Lipoprotein lipase is the enzyme with this activity.

3 **True** Lipoprotein lipase hydrolyses 90% of chylomicron triglycerides to free fatty acids which are re-esterified to form fat droplets in adipocytes.

4 **False** Coronary heart disease accounts for ≈30% of deaths in men and 25% of deaths in women.

5 **True** High density lipoprotein (HDL) scavenges redundant tissue cholesterol and returns it to the liver.

Case 13

1 **True** Direct involvement of the heart muscle itself is an important cause of heart failure. It is responsible for death during the acute stage of the disease as well as for morbidity in later life.

2 **False** Although the deposition of fibrin on the surface of the heart can be extensive and can even calcify, pericardial constriction does not occur.

3 **True** The progression of dilated cardiomyopathy caused by prolonged, excessive alcohol consumption may be halted or even reversed by abstinence.

4 **False** High output cardiac failure is a

classical but rare association of Paget's disease, and only occurs when over one-third of the skeleton is involved.

5 **False** Sinus tachycardia with or without extrasystoles is almost invariably present. In chronic cases, atrial fibrillation is also commonly found.

Case 14

1 **False** Dressler's syndrome, thought to be an autoimmune-mediated pericarditis, pleuritis and/or pneumonitis, develops up to 6 weeks after myocardial infarction.
2 **True** The earlier the treatment, the more dramatic the benefit.
3 **True** Emboli from left ventricular mural thrombus can traverse the coronary ostia, particularly if ejected at the end of systole, and obstruct other coronary vessels.
4 **True** Preservation of ischaemic myocardium, that might otherwise have died and been rendered electrically inert, may predispose to dysrhythmias.
5 **True** The incidence of this once common complication continues to decline as the 'pain onset to needle time' declines.

Case 15

1 **False** Sudden death occurs in 2% of patients and 10% have a myocardial infarction.
2 **False** An increase in myocardial oxygen demand precipitates stable angina. Unstable angina, like myocardial infarction, is brought about by a reduction in myocardial oxygen supply.
3 **False** Walking uphill, cold weather, anxiety and eating rather than fasting tend to precipitate angina.
4 **False** The mechanism is a rare cause of ischaemia, sometimes known as variant or Prinzmetal's angina.
5 **False** Coronary atherosclerosis is often present before the age of 20 years.

Case 16

1 **True** Mitral or aortic valve vegetations can embolize and be forced down the coronary artery ostia.
2 **False** Destruction of the valves necessitates urgent surgical intervention irrespective of ongoing infection.
3 **True** Oral temperatures between 37.2 and 35.8 °C can safely be regarded as normal.
4 **True** The progesterone-induced increase in core temperature is used as a test of ovulation as the progesterone-producing corpus luteum is not formed until ovulation has occurred.
5 **True** This polypeptide product of monocytes and macrophages has many effects, including an increase in body temperature to a new set point.

Case 17

1 **True** The prevalence of atrial fibrillation increases from 0.5% of patients under 60 years to 4% of those over 60 years and to over 10% of those over 75 years.
2 **False** Atrial fibrillation is associated with thyrotoxicosis rather than hypothyroidism. The association with mitral stenosis is of course true.
3 **False** The usual reduction in cardiac output is around 10%. Although the difference in cardiac output may appear relatively trivial, the improvement in patients' wellbeing after successful cardioversion is often dramatic.
4 **True** A number of major placebo-controlled trials have shown that the 66% reduction in thromboembolic events more than outweighs the small risk of major haemorrhage (0.3% per year).
5 **True** Treated with placebo only, 35% of cases of atrial fibrillation of short duration cardiovert spontaneously within 6 h and, within 8 h, up to 48% of cases spontaneously revert to sinus rhythm.

Case 18

1 **False** Polycystic renal disease is an autosomal dominant condition that is responsible for around 10% of cases of end-stage chronic renal failure.
2 **True** Subarachnoid haemorrhage from intracranial aneurysms is the cause of death in 9% of patients with polycystic renal disease.
3 **False** Hepatic cysts are present in 30% of patients, but hepatic function is usually preserved.
4 **True** The plot of the reciprocal serum creatinine level against time does predict terminal renal failure and the requirement for dialysis.
5 **True** Careful dietary protein restriction slows the progression of chronic renal failure.

Case 19

1 **True** Calcium salts, uric acid and mixtures of magnesium and ammonium phosphates account for almost all renal stones produced.
2 **False** Many renal stones are discovered completely incidentally on plain abdominal X-ray taken for other reasons.
3 **False** They tend to be struvite, a mixture of magnesium and ammonium phosphates.
4 **False** Unfortunately not. The tendency does not wane.
5 **False** The association is with hypercalciuria rather than hypercalcaemia.

Case 20

1 **False** Lung cancer is now more common than breast cancer as a cause of death in women. Lung cancer also kills 7% of males who smoke.
2 **False** Although partly reversible, chronic obstructive pulmonary disease (COPD) is a slowly progressive airways' disorder that remains, by definition, fairly stable over time. Steroid-induced reversibility is a feature of asthma rather than COPD.
3 **True** At this level of forced expiratory volume the condition is classified as severe.
4 **False** The figure is in fact closer to 50%.
5 **True** An improvement in the forced expiratory volume in 1 s (FEV1) of 15% or 200 mL suggests an element of bronchospasm.

Case 21

1 **False** The pressure in the thorax remains below atmospheric pressure. If it equalled atmospheric pressure, the elastic recoil of the lungs would make them collapse.
2 **False** The pleura is derived from the mesoderm.
3 **True** This is a common false localizing sign.
4 **True** It is resorbed by the visceral pleura.
5 **False** The pain is usually sharp, localized and exacerbated by deep inspiration.

Case 22

1 **False** As perfusion of the affected, hypoventilated area continues, an effective right to left shunt develops which decreases P_aO_2.
2 **True** As the compliance of the lung decreases, reduced tidal volume and increased respiratory rate become the most energy-effective pattern of breathing even in the absence of the constraints imposed by pleuritic pain.
3 **True** Other organisms include *Pneumocystis carinii* and *Cryptococcus neoformans*, as well as more typical organisms.
4 **True** Fortunately, the majority of infections do not result in overt disease.
5 **False** Most patients who comply with treatment are rendered non-infectious within 2 weeks of the start of chemotherapy.

Case 23

1 **False** There is no pathological distinction between the 'blue bloater' and 'pink puffer' phenotypes.
2 **True** Particles larger than this are not carried to the alveoli, and particles smaller than this remain in suspension and are exhaled.
3 **False** The latent period after asbestos exposure is 15–19 years.
4 **False** The effect is synergistic, unlike the risk of mesothelioma, which is not increased by concurrent smoking.
5 **True** Farmer's lung is a relatively common extrinsic allergic alveolitis caused by inhalation of the spores of thermophilic actinomycetes found in mouldy hay, straw or grain.

Case 24

1 **True** Blood gas markers of a very severe attack are acidosis, an oxygen saturation of less than 92%, normal or high P_aCO_2 (5–6 kPa, 36–45 mmHg) and severe hypoxia $P_aO_2 < 8$ kPa (60 mmHg) irrespective of concurrent oxygen treatment.
2 **False** Sedation is dangerous in asthma attacks.
3 **False** Even though the partial pressure of oxygen in the blood falls by this amount, saturation decreases by only 4–5%.
4 **True** A reduced forced expiratory volume in 1 s (FEV1) and increased functional residual capacity are often present.
5 **False** Hypoxaemia is an invariable feature of asthma attacks.

Case 25

1 **False** Although the histological changes are often present at that time, significant proteinuria usually takes 15 years to develop.
2 **False** Unfortunately, these end points occur within 5 years and, if proteinuria is heavy (>5 g per 24 h), the mortality at 2 years is 50%.
3 **False** They are relatively trivial causes. The main causes are diabetes in the developed world and cataract, trachoma and river blindness in developing countries.
4 **False** Over the first year, improvements in diabetic control may be associated with a slight increase in the rate of progression of retinopathy. After that time, progression is markedly slowed and this more than makes up for the initial changes. Risks of nephropathy and neuropathy are also reduced.
5 **False** The risk in insulin-dependent diabetes is <4% for first degree relatives, compared with 25% in non-insulin-dependent diabetes.

Case 26

1 **True** Increase in size of the hands and feet can be so subtle that the significance of changing shoe and glove size is not recognized by the patient.
2 **False** Classically, the ulnar innervation to the fifth finger and part of the ring finger is spared.
3 **True** Changes in occlusion are common, and predispose towards arthritis of the temporomandibular joint.
4 **True** Many causes have been postulated, including increased plasma volume and total body sodium levels, inappropriate activation of the renin–angiotensin system or a direct action of growth hormone or insulin-like growth factor 1 (IGF-1) at the kidneys, causing sodium retention.
5 **False** In almost all cases, the effects of growth hormone hypersecretion lead to the diagnosis being made before the somatotrophic adenoma reaches a size that would impinge on the optic chiasm.

Case 27

1 **False** In most circumstances, the presence

of a spontaneous fracture with no other cause found is evidence enough of 'established osteoporosis'.

2 **False** Bone is remodelled at about 10% per annum. Areas of bone under high stress can be remodelled much faster, and a rate of 18% per year is not unusual.

3 **False** Genetics is the most important determining factor of osteoporotic risk. Approximately 85% of lumbar bone density is heritable.

4 **True** Typical markers of bone formation are alkaline phosphatase (bone isoenzyme) and a timed urine collection for osteocalcin.

5 **True** Parathyroid hormone enhances calcium absorption and increases phosphate loss from the kidneys, stimulates the activity of osteoclasts causing efflux of calcium and phosphate from the skeleton and stimulates 1α-hydroxylase activity in the proximal tubular cells which enhances production of activated vitamin D.

Case 28

1 **True** A series of iodinated proteins is formed by this process, the most prevalent being thyroglobulin.

2 **False** Monoiodotyrosine and diiodotyrosine are coupled together to form the active thyroid hormones triiodothyronine (T3) and thyroxine.

3 **False** These symptoms, although classically associated with Graves' disease, are very rare.

4 **False** Lid lag is failure of the upper lid to begin its descent simultaneously with the globe on downward gaze.

5 **False** Lid retraction—a visible rim of sclera above the cornea—is a feature of the sympathetic overactivity that occurs in thyrotoxicosis. Unlike proptosis (forward movement of the globe caused by infiltrative ophthalmopathy) and periorbital oedema, it is not one of the specific features of Graves' ophthalmopathy.

Case 29

1 **False** It is the lack of insulin that leads to a rapid rise in hepatic glucose output and a fall in peripheral glucose uptake.

2 **False** Starvation and alcohol can both cause ketonuria and alcohol can cause ketoacidosis. In ketoacidosis, ketone bodies are elevated in the blood and urine, in association with a metabolic acidosis.

3 **False** This is not possible. Insulin and rehydration with saline are essential elements in the treatment of this condition.

4 **False** Vomiting is largely brought about by contraction of the diaphragm and abdominal musculature and relaxation of the gastric fundus.

5 **True** One of the signs of anorexia nervosa, in which the patient tends to induce repeated vomiting after eating to avoid weight gain, is marked etching of dental enamel due to gastric acid exposure.

Case 30

1 **False** Hyperglycaemia, the biochemical characteristic of insulin-dependent diabetes, starts as the autoimmune destruction of insulin-producing cells—the pathological process of the disease—reaches its end.

2 **True** Sympathetic activity suppresses insulin release and increases glucagon release during exercise.

3 **False** In most if not all cases, diabetes mellitus can be diagnosed on the basis of a fasting or random blood glucose level.

4 **True** There is thought to be extensive cross-talk between the various cellular subtypes within the pancreatic islets. The increased circulating levels of glucagon in diabetes are thought to be related to local insulin privation.

5 **False** Approximately 80% of the cells are insulin producing.

Case 31

1 **False** Although some degree of axonal damage may occur, the mechanism of Guillain–Barré syndrome is predominantly an acute immune-mediated demyelinating polyneuropathy.
2 **False** The syndrome usually develops within 2 weeks and always within 4 weeks of the infection.
3 **False** Respiratory, bulbar and extraocular muscles are not infrequently involved. Close monitoring of patients is critical as involvement of these muscles prevents the patient from calling for help. Approximately 25% of patients need respiratory support.
4 **False** 15% of patients have residual disability.
5 **True** They can produce adenosine triphosphate (ATP) quickly from glycogen by anaerobic glycolysis, but the formation of lactic acid leads rapidly to muscle fatigue.

Case 32

1 **False** Involvement of the ophthalmic division of the trigeminal nerve is rare, particularly in isolation.
2 **False** Sensory loss cannot normally be demonstrated.
3 **True** The whole episode of attacks of trigeminal neuralgia tends to resolve after a few weeks, but may subsequently recur.
4 **True** This symptom often occurs in young women and is localized to one cheek.
5 **True** Severe pain in the eye is often felt to radiate back into the head.

Case 33

1 **True** Both simple and complex partial seizures can generalize with loss of consciousness and convulsive motor activity.
2 **False** The presence of an aura or focal feature before the onset of a convulsion is an important pointer towards a focal rather than a primary generalized seizure.
3 **False** The electroencephalogram (EEG) does show a pathognomonic 3-Hz spike and wave discharges, but these occur synchronously throughout all the leads.
4 **True** One-third of patients outgrow them, one-third continue to have simple absence seizures and one-third go on to occasional concomitant generalized tonic–clonic seizures.
5 **True** This is true. However, seizures occurring between 1 and 14 days after central nervous system injury indicate a high likelihood of post-traumatic epilepsy.

Case 34

1 **True** This distinguishes their activity from that of the primary motor cortex.
2 **False** Tremor, bradykinesia and muscular rigidity are more typical signs. Weakness results from damage to the upper or lower motor neurones.
3 **False** Unfortunately, the underlying degenerative processes continue unabated and, in many cases, render the medication less and less effective with time.
4 **False** Anticholinergic drugs are often more effective in relieving tremor. The primary function of dopamine is to relieve bradykinesia.
5 **False** So-called lead pipe rigidity, which remains constant throughout the range of movement, is typical. Clasp-knife rigidity, which is less evident at the very beginning and towards the end of the movement, is typical of corticospinal lesions.

Case 35

1 **True** Also, ≈40% of patients with multiple sclerosis develop optic neuritis at some time.
2 **False** The demyelination in multiple sclerosis is characteristically asymmetrical.
3 **True** This is the fascicle in the brain stem

that connects the IIIrd, IVth and VIth cranial nerve nuclei.

4 **False** Spinal cord involvement in demyelination produces upper motor neurone signs.

5 **False** Ipsilateral signs are produced. The effects of cerebellar involvement in disease are complex, and sometimes even fairly extensive lesions produce very little in the way of clinical signs.

Case 36

1 **False** Although patients often complain that the face feels 'numb', there is never any objective evidence of facial sensory loss in Bell's palsy as the Vth nerve remains intact.

2 **False** A complete recovery is seen in only 60% of patients. As many as 20% of patients are left with marked facial asymmetry.

3 **False** The facial nerve closes the eye. The IIIrd nerve and sympathetic supply are predominantly responsible for opening it.

4 **False** Sensory innervation, with the exception of taste, is mediated by the Vth cranial nerve. The facial nerve subserves taste sensation to this region.

5 **True** In lower motor neurone facial palsy, sounds may seem excessively loud owing to paralysis of the stapedius muscle which, under normal circumstances, reflexly damps vibration of the tympanic membrane.

Case 37

1 **True** There is also a 2–3% annual risk of myocardial infarction. The combined risk of vascular death after a transient ischaemic attack (TIA) is 9% over the first year, with the greatest risk being in the first 3 months, then about 6% per year for the next 5 years.

2 **False** This would be exceptionally unusual. The signs are usually weakness of the whole or part of one side of the body, with numbness rather than tingling if sensory symptoms are evident.

3 **False** The carotid territory is affected in 80% of TIAs, producing unilateral weakness or sensory loss, monocular visual loss or aphasia.

4 **False** Trials show that surgically treated patients do better at 2 and 3 years, although there is an increased morbidity and mortality associated with surgery in the first 3 months.

5 **False** The sympathetic nerve fibres run dorsolaterally in the brain stem.

Case 38

1 **True** Of the 0.2% of the population who suffer a stroke annually in Europe, 80% are ischaemic and 20% haemorrhagic.

2 **True** Analysis of studies carried out to examine the relationship between lipid-lowering drugs and cardiovascular disease indicate that, in addition to a reduction in the risk of a fatal heart attack of over 30%, treatment with statins (HMGCoA-reductase inhibitors) results in a 24% decrease in fatal and non-fatal stroke.

3 **False** Dysphasia results from damage to the dominant hemisphere. Dyspraxia, loss of skilled motor activities such as feeding or dressing, results from damage to the non-dominant parietal lobe.

4 **True** The same pattern can be produced by anterior choroidal artery occlusion and by haemorrhage into the internal capsule.

5 **False** Sensory and visual defects are characteristic.

Case 39

1 **True** The type III immune complex allergic mechanism is thought to be a form of panniculitis. Panniculitis is inflammation of the fat. Lipodystrophy is genetically mediated fat wasting, and lipoatrophy and lipohypertrophy are local problems associated with repeated subcutaneous injection of insulin.

2 **False** They are less oxidized than proteins and carbohydrates; hence, their ability to be extensively oxidized to release energy. In addition, being hydrophobic, they can be stored in an almost anhydrous form.
3 **False** Typically, fat stores contain enough energy to last for several months.
4 **False** 5α-Reductase converts testosterone to the more potent androgen dihydrotestosterone. Adipose tissue contains aromatase, which converts preandrogens to testosterone and to oestrone.
5 **False** There is no dietary requirement for cholesterol. However, humans lack the enzymes to introduce double bonds distal to C-9 in fatty acids, and therefore require dietary linoleate and linolenate.

Case 40

1 **False** Over 50% of patients have the histocompatibility antigen HLA-DW4. HLA-B27 is associated with ankylosing spondylitis and other ankylosing spondarthropathies.
2 **False** Heberden's nodes, osteophytic enlargement around the distal interphalangeal joints, are characteristic of osteoarthritis.
3 **True** Episcleritis is a rare complication of rheumatoid disease.
4 **True** Sutures join the bones of the skull, syndesmoses join bones such as the tibia and fibula and gomphoses attach the teeth to their alveolar sockets.
5 **False** The joints between the shaft and epiphyses of long bones are cartilaginous, not synovial.

Case 41

1 **True** Around 10–15% of symptomatically hyperuricaemic patients have a family history of gout. On careful questioning about symptoms and signs, the figures are considerably higher.
2 **False** Although patients with gout have been hyperuricaemic at some time, persistent hyperuricaemia is unusual. Conversely, 18% of the population have hyperuricaemia, yet relatively few suffer attacks of gout.
3 **True** The absence of crystals after careful examination makes the diagnosis unlikely.
4 **True** The association with obesity is particularly strong.
5 **True** In addition, at least half of all initial attacks involve the great toe and 90% of initial attacks present as a monoarthritis.

Case 42

1 **True** It is, and a raised ferritin level is found in untreated haemochromatosis. As ferritin is an acute phase protein, however, the specificity of a normal or raised ferritin level is much lower than that of a very low level.
2 **True** The carrier frequency is almost 10% and the disease affects 0.3% of the population.
3 **True** It is caused by deposition of iron in the pituitary gland and in the testes themselves.
4 **False** The pigmentation is melanin.
5 **False** As free iron is toxic, it is transported loosely bound to transferrin and stored intracellularly as the protein complexes ferritin and haemosiderin.

Case 43

1 **False** Serum ferritin closely correlates with total body iron stores. While levels below the normal range are diagnostic of iron deficiency, serum ferritin can be falsely elevated into the normal range despite iron deficiency as it is an acute phase protein.
2 **True** Gluten-induced enteropathy is one of the most common causes of malabsorption in the UK population.
3 **True** Dermatitis herpetiformis is characterized by an itchy, blistering rash

that affects the back, buttocks, elbows and knees. It does improve with exclusion of gluten from the diet.

4 **False** Most of the toxicity of gliadins is expended in the upper small intestine as the gluten is hydrolysed to a less toxic form during its progress distally.

5 **True** There is a 10-fold increased risk of gastrointestinal tumours and a 40-fold increased risk of intestinal lymphoma in coeliac disease which returns to normal 5 years after gluten is excluded from the diet.

Case 44

1 **False** It starts at the rectum and extends proximally to involve part or all of the large intestine.

2 **True** 10% of patients have a first degree relative with the condition.

3 **False** In general, food residue remains in the colon for between 12 h and 3 days while relatively small amounts of water, salts and water-soluble vitamins are absorbed.

4 **False** Bile salts are usually reabsorbed in the terminal ileum. Their ingress into the colon produces bile salt-induced enteropathy.

5 **False** The mechanism of intermittent diarrhoea in irritable bowel syndrome is decreased absorption. Secretory diarrhoea is typical of bile salt-induced enteropathy, and exudative diarrhoea is typical of ulcerative colitis.

Case 45

1 **True** Transamination is also the synthetic route of most non-essential amino acids.

2 **True** In most cases, the infection is associated with chronic fatigue rather than jaundice.

3 **True** The liver is largely responsible for controlling levels of circulating blood sugar.

4 **False** Permanent memory impairment can be one of the most difficult aspects for reformed alcoholics to cope with.

5 **False** Very few patients become virus free.

Case 46

1 **True** Without thiamine (vitamin B_1), pyruvate cannot be oxidized to acetyl-coenzyme A, glucose cannot be utilized aerobically and pyruvic and lactic acids accumulate.

2 **True** The presence of carbohydrate increases the amounts of pyruvate and lactate that accumulate, and leads to high output cardiac failure and oedema characteristic of 'wet' beriberi.

3 **False** Pellagra is caused by nicotinic acid (nicotinamide) deficiency.

4 **False** The tear involves the mucosa only. Bleeding can nevertheless be quite severe, but healing is usually rapid.

5 **True** Petechial haemorrhages affect the upper midbrain (superior colliculi). Ophthalmoplegia is one of the most characteristic clinical findings.

Case 47

1 **True** The mechanism of this effect is unclear.

2 **True** The diagnosis is made by identifying urease action in biopsy specimens or ^{13}C- or ^{14}C-tagged carbon dioxide in the breath after ingestion of a bolus of ^{14}C urea. One of the mechanisms used by *Helicobacter pylori* to protect itself from the acid environment of the stomach is to convert urea into ammonia which forms alkaline ammonium hydroxide in solution.

3 **False** It is a Gram-negative bacterium.

4 **True** Eradication of the organism is associated with a cure of the disease in most patients.

5 **True** Remarkably, lymphoma regression occurs in a high proportion of patients after *H. pylori* eradication.

Case 48

1 **True** In many patients with impaired but stable hepatic function, infections, drugs or surgical procedures themselves may lead to encephalopathy which is often reversible. The condition can, however, be chronic, progressive and lead to death.
2 **True** Severe hepatic dysfunction and/or extrahepatic or intrahepatic shunting of portal blood into the systemic circulation is a prerequisite for the development of hepatic encephalopathy.
3 **True** Alkalosis increases lipid-soluble ammonia (NH_3) at the expense of ammonium ions (NH_4^+). Ammonia is more able to cross the blood–brain barrier.
4 **False** The rate of metabolism remains at about 10 g (1 unit) per hour irrespective of plasma concentrations.
5 **True** So does rapid gastric emptying, the absence of food and dilution to 20% by volume.

Case 49

1 **False** Porphyrins are compounds produced during the synthesis rather than the catabolism of haemoglobin. Bilirubin is the product of haemoglobin catabolism.
2 **False** Pale stools and dark urine are signs associated with obstructive jaundice.
3 **False** Conjugated bilirubin is either excreted unchanged or metabolized to urobilinogen through the action of bacteria in the lower small intestine and colon, and partially reabsorbed into the portal circulation.
4 **True** About 15% of bilirubin is derived from the direct destruction of maturing red cells in the bone marrow.
5 **True** As urobilinogen is formed in the gut and reabsorbed from the lower small intestine and colon, its presence in the urine must indicate flow of bilirubin into the gut, a process that depends on prior conjugation.

Case 50

1 **False** The diarrhoea is intermittent, and often punctuated by episodic constipation.
2 **True** Irritable bowel disease is not associated with constant abdominal pain or distension, constant diarrhoea, weight loss or the passage of blood with stool. In this case, the blood was from a prolapsed haemorrhoid.
3 **False** Personality disorders occur in 60% of patients presenting with parasuicide. Unfortunately, borderline personality disorder does not respond well to psychotherapy.
4 **False** This is a very characteristic symptom of irritable bowel syndrome.
5 **True** On direct questioning, the majority of people have at least one symptom associated with irritable bowel syndrome. At least 13% of women and 5% of men have three or more of these symptoms.

Index

Note:
Index entries on pages 137–148 refer to the answers of the MCQs, but index references are only included if information is provided that is not discussed in the case history.
Page numbers in **bold** refer to the diagnosis and main features of the case history.

Instructions for use of CD

1 Install the CD according to the instructions given in the booklet.
2 First screen: select whether you want to view the cases randomly (click central icon) or by system (click desired system icon).
3 Play the video clip(s).
4 Think about the differential diagnosis.
5 Look at the case notes in the book and read the basic science associated with the case. Note that the case resolution and basic science are NOT included on the CD, they are only in the book.
6 Try the multiple choice questions either on the CD or in the book.
7 The bottom left icon reveals useful diagrams for you to look at. (These are often extra diagrams that do not appear in the book.)

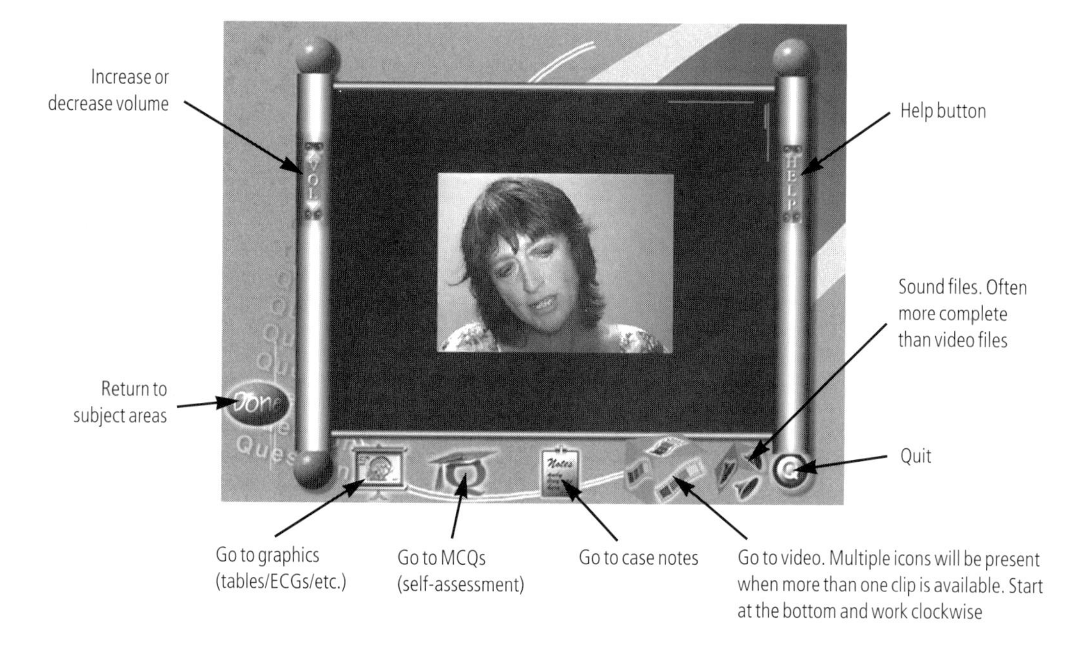

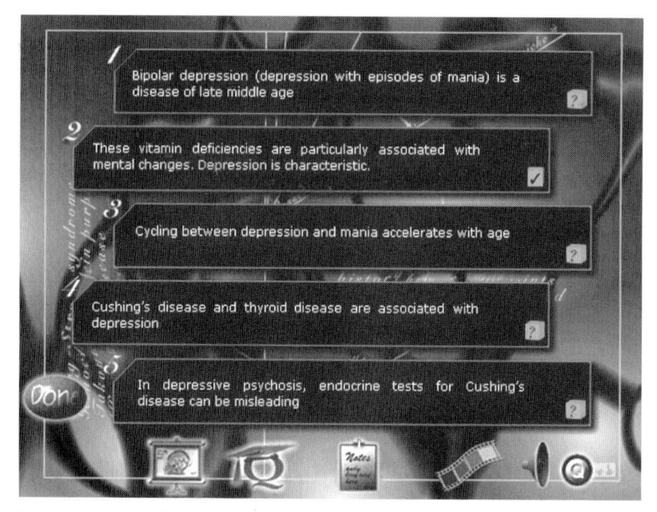

Self-assessment — True/False questions